Strength & Power for Young Athletes

Avery D. Faigenbaum, EdD

University of Massachusetts–Boston

Wayne L. Westcott, PhD

South Shore YMCA
Quincy, Massachusetts

Human Kinetics

Library of Congress Cataloging-in-Publication Data

Faigenbaum, Avery D., 1961-
    Strength & power for young athletes / Avery D. Faigenbaum and Wayne L. Westcott.
        p. cm.
    Includes index.
    ISBN 0-7360-0218-9
        1. Exercise for children.   2. Physical fitness for children.   I. Title: Strength and power
    for young athletes.   II. Westcott, Wayne L. 1949-   III. Title.
RJ133.F35   2000
613.7'042--dc21   99-089903
                                                                                              CIP

ISBN: 0-7360-0218-9

Acquisitions Editor: Martin Barnard; **Developmental Editor**: Patricia Norris; **Assistant Editors**: Wendy McLaughlin, Melissa Feld, Derek Campbell, and Laura Majersky; **Copyeditor**: Danelle Eknes; **Proofreader**: Kathy Bennett; **Indexer**: Betty Frizzell; **Permissions Manager**: Cheri Banks; **Graphic Designer**: Robert Reuther; **Graphic Artist**: Sandra Meier; **Photo Editor:** Clark Brooks**; Cover Designer**: Keith Blomberg; **Photographer (cover)**: Tom Roberts; **Photographer (interior)**: Tom Roberts**; Printer**: Versa Press

Human Kinetics books are available at special discounts for bulk purchase. Special editions or book excerpts can also be created to specification. For details, contact the Special Sales Manager at Human Kinetics.

Printed in the United States of America

10   9   8   7   6   5   4   3   2   1

Human Kinetics
Web site: http://www.humankinetics.com/

United States: Human Kinetics
P.O. Box 5076, Champaign, IL 61825-5076
1-800-747-4457
e-mail: humank@hkusa.com

Canada: Human Kinetics
475 Devonshire Road Unit 100, Windsor, ON N8Y 2L5
1-800-465-7301 (in Canada only)
e-mail: humank@hkcanada.com

Europe: Human Kinetics
P.O. Box IW14, Leeds LS16 6TR, United Kingdom
+44 (0)113-278 1708
e-mail: humank@hkeurope.com

Australia: Human Kinetics
57A Price Avenue, Lower Mitcham, South Australia 5062
(08) 82771555
e-mail: liahka@senet.com.au

New Zealand: Human Kinetics
P.O. Box 105-231, Auckland Central
09-523-3462
e-mail: humank@hknewz.com

It is with great appreciation that we dedicate this book to the hundreds of boys and girls who have participated so enthusiastically in our strength-training programs, and to their most accommodating parents who have clearly understood the value of developing a strong musculoskeletal system at a young age for a lifetime full of physical activity and personal fitness.

CONTENTS

Foreword vi

Acknowledgments vii

Introduction viii

PART I   Strength Development   1

Chapter 1   **Ready to Train**   3

Chapter 2   **Program Prescriptions**   9

Chapter 3   **Correct Technique and Injury Prevention**   . . 21

Chapter 4   **Eating for Strength** 27

PART II   Equipment and Exercise   37

Chapter 5   **Free Weights**   39

Chapter 6   **Weight Machines** 71

Chapter 7   Cords and Balls 93

Chapter 8   Body-Weight Exercises 121

PART III   Age-Group Strength Programs   137

Chapter 9   Mighty Mites: 7- to 9-Year-Olds 139

Chapter 10   Junior Builders: 10- to 12-Year-Olds 145

Chapter 11   Teens of Steel: 13- to 15-Year-Olds 151

PART IV   Strength Programs for Sports   159

Chapter 12   General Sport-Conditioning Programs . . . 161

Chapter 13   Power Sports 173
             Football, Rugby, Wrestling, Gymnastics, Track and Field

Chapter 14   Jumping Sports 177
             Basketball, Volleyball, Netball, Dance, Figure Skating

Chapter 15   Striking Sports 181
             Baseball, Softball, Tennis, Hockey, Golf

Chapter 16   Endurance Sports 187
             Soccer, Field Hockey, Lacrosse, Cross Country, Swimming

Appendix A: Free Weights 193
Appendix B: Weight Machines 197
Index 200
About the Authors 204

Foreword

It gives me great pleasure to provide a foreword for a book that covers such important subject matter written by two gentlemen whose careers and research I have followed with interest.

Once a controversial field with many detractors, strength training for children and adolescents is now coming to be recognized for what it is—an indispensable part of any young athlete's workout regimen. Erroneous concerns about the safety and effectiveness of strength training for young people have been dispelled thanks in part to the efforts of researchers such as Dr. Westcott and Dr. Faigenbaum. Indeed, more people than ever before understand that it's safe for kids to train with weights, and also that young athletes who train with weights not only perform better, but are also less likely to get injured.

I am especially impressed by this book because it expertly combines theory with practice. The material in these pages will satisfy anyone who wants to know the principles of strength training and the science behind them. It is also a terrific "how-to" resource for adults who intend to train young athletes to build strength with weights.

I cannot recommend this book highly enough to sportscare professionals such as coaches and athletic trainers and interested members of the lay public—parents, especially—who want to learn more about strength training for children and adolescents.

Lyle J. Micheli, MD
Director—Sports Medicine Division, Boston Children's Hospital
Past President, American College of Sports Medicine

Acknowledgments

It is a great privilege to acknowledge the many gifted individuals who so generously gave of their time and talents in helping us produce this book. We are most grateful for the professional leadership at Human Kinetics, and especially appreciate the expert assistance from our Acquisitions Editor, Martin Barnard, our Developmental Editor, Pat Norris, and our assistant editor, Wendy McLaughlin. We believe this book has outstanding exercise illustrations, and we sincerely thank Tom Roberts for his superb photography skills in making this possible. We are indebted to Debra Wein, MS, RD, our nutrition consultant, for her most pertinent professional advice in this area. We are particularly pleased with Susan Ramsden's expertise in writing portions of the youth nutrition chapter. We also thank Susan for her excellent work in typing our original texts and designing our original tables, figures, and charts. We congratulate all of our youth strength-training class members who demonstrated correct exercise technique for the photos, as well as our fine teenage models, Jennifer Pizzi, Zachary Smith, and Matt Yohe.

We are most grateful to Rita La Rosa Loud for her innovative leadership in our youth strength-training classes, and to all of the youth who have participated in this unique fitness program. Finally, we deeply appreciate the support of the South Shore YMCA President, Ralph Yohe; Vice President, Mary Moore; and Executive Director, William Johnson; as well as the Nautilus Director, Claudia Westcott; and the Fitness Directors, Gayle Laing, Cindy Long, and Tish Holmes for their unswerving support of our youth strength-training program. We also appreciate the many student interns who have provided outstanding instruction and supervision to our class participants. We are most grateful to Dr. Lyle Micheli and his sports medicine staff at Boston Children's Hospital, for performing physical examinations on children in our research studies. Finally, we thank God for over 15 years of safe and successful youth strength-training experiences, and for all of the parents who have entrusted their children to our exercise program.

Introduction

We have something in common. We want to help young people become physically fit so they can enjoy an active lifestyle and success in sports. We want to turn the tide on sedentary lifestyles by presenting boys and girls with safe and sensible strength-training programs that will help them look good, feel good, and function well at home, in school, and on the athletic field.

We know that even naturally energetic children have many temptations toward inactivity, such as television, movies, videos, computers, and similar sedentary pursuits. The eventual result is an undesirable body composition (fat-to-muscle ratio) and poor sport performance. Unfortunately, youth who are underfit and overfat typically become adults who are underfit and overfat, which increases their risk for injury, illness, and premature death.

So what can we do to reverse the trend toward inactivity among our children? We believe that the first and most important step is to help them develop a functional musculoskeletal system. Boys and girls should have strong muscles, bones, tendons, and ligaments that enable them to perform physical activities with a high level of success and a low risk of injury. Muscles are the engines of the body, and most young people can benefit from more powerful engines. At last report, only one out of two American children could perform a single pull-up. This finding reveals serious upper-body weakness and partly explains why so many boys and girls avoid the physical activities they should be enjoying during their childhood. Even if your child gets on base every time he or she bats, why settle for singles, when stronger muscles could result in doubles, triples, and home runs?

The best means for building musculoskeletal strength is progressive resistance exercise. More commonly known as strength training, progressive resistance exercise requires muscles to produce force against appropriate weight loads (or other types of resistance), which you increase gradually as the musculoskeletal system becomes stronger. Part I, chapters 1, 2, and 3, presents the basic strength-training benefits, guidelines, and program considerations, while chapter 4 focuses on proper nutrition for young exercisers.

The recommended program of progressive resistance exercise is highly effective for increasing muscle strength, and it is much less stressful (both physically and mentally) than trying to do a few pull-ups, push-ups, or bar dips with an unchangeable body weight. Over the past 15 years we have conducted dozens of strength-training programs with hundreds of boys and girls between 6 and 15 years of age. All participants achieved significant strength gains and none experienced a training-related injury. On average, the youth who completed our eight-week exercise program increased their muscle strength by about 60 percent, although some training protocols have proved more productive than others. We present equipment options and exercise techniques in part II, chapters 5, 6, 7, and 8. Part III, chapters 9, 10, and 11, provides three age-appropriate strength-training programs and research-based training recommendations for children 7 to 9 years, 10 to 12 years, and 13 to 15 years.

Our youth strength-training studies have also shown significant improvements in the participants' body composition. Although growing boys and girls gain lean weight (muscle, bone, etc.) through normal maturation processes, those who do strength exercise are more likely to experience favorable changes in body composition than those who do not strength train.

Another positive outcome of youth strength training is greater self-esteem in the boys and girls who complete the program. As their muscle strength increases, so does their self-confidence. Our research indicates that, in addition to feeling better about themselves, many young people are willing to try other physical activities (team sports, rock climbing, swimming, etc.) following successful strength-training experiences.

Strength training can also facilitate beneficial lifestyle changes in previously sedentary children. In our school-based study with unfit and overweight fifth grade students, 96 percent reported more out-of-school exercise activity and 100 percent reported better eating habits as a result of the strength-training program.

Strength training is an ideal physical activity for overweight boys and girls. Although their excess weight works against them in endurance exercise such as running, soccer, and basketball, it works for them in strength training. Heavier children generally use more resistance than lighter children, which tends to increase their status in the weight room. Strength training also helps them burn excess calories, both during exercise sessions and following the training session, due to its elevating effect on metabolic rate.

Well-designed youth strength-training programs typically foster positive social interaction and cooperation among the participants. Consider training boys and girls in pairs so partners can encourage each other, offer feedback on form, and provide assistance if necessary.

For those young people involved in athletic activities, strength training is important to reduce the risk of muscle imbalance and overuse injuries. In fact, according to the American College of Sports Medicine, children could prevent over 50 percent of their sport-training injuries by participating in physical-conditioning programs that include strength exercise.

In addition to its key role in injury reduction, a strong musculoskeletal system can enhance sport performance in young athletes. Let's take the example of strength training for girls cross country runners. It is a fact that the female cross country runners have the highest injury rate of all interscholastic sports teams, including football and gymnastics. Now, consider the results of our strength-training study with the Notre Dame High School cross country team. For four consecutive years, these young female athletes did 30 minutes of strength exercise, three days a week, during the summer and winter months. Over the entire four-year period, only one runner experienced an injury, indicating that the strength-training program was a highly effective injury deterrent. Perhaps even more impressive, during the same four years these cross country runners won four consecutive New England team championships.

These and similar results with other boys' and girls' sports teams clearly indicate that strong muscles have a positive effect on athletic performance. For this reason, we dedicated part four of this book to sport-specific strength-training programs. Chapter 12 provides the basic conditioning program for all youth sport participants, whereas chapters 13, 14, 15, and 16 present clearly defined exercise protocols for five power sports, five jumping sports, five striking sports, and five endurance sports.

So strength training may help young people increase muscle strength, improve body composition, enhance self-esteem, increase physical activity, improve eating habits, develop cooperation skills, avoid athletic injuries, and enhance sport performance. To the best of our knowledge, there are no negative consequences associated with a sensible and supervised youth strength-training program. However, just as you wouldn't give children skis and send them up the mountain alone, you shouldn't give youth a weight set and expect them to use it safely and productively. Careful and competent instruction is *the most important factor* in successful strength exercise for young people.

The primary purpose of this book is to help you develop the essential knowledge and teaching skills to safely and effectively instruct youth strength-training programs. The chapters that follow present research-based principles and practical applications for implementing an age-appropriate strength-training program for preteens and teens. We carefully describe and illustrate a variety of resistance exercises using machines, free weights, bands, and body weight. We provide sample sport-specific strength-training protocols along with recommended aerobic activities and stretching exercises to ensure overall fitness development. We believe that this book provides all the tools you need to become competent and confident in teaching sensible strength training to boys and girls.

PART I

Strength Development

1

Ready to Train

You've picked up this book on youth strength training, so you are at least interested in this topic. In fact, you probably have some knowledge about strength training, and your intuition tells you that supervised strength exercise should be good for boys and girls, especially because they typically do little muscle-conditioning activity.

However, you've also heard that children should not train with weights because it either doesn't work, places too much stress on growing muscles, or is dangerous. Categorically, all these misperceptions are untrue. As you are undoubtedly aware, strength-building exercise can be highly beneficial to growing boys and girls. However, because children are not miniature adults, you must progress cautiously when training young people. Over the past several years, research has clearly demonstrated that strength exercise is a safe, effective, and efficient means for conditioning young muscles, as long as certain safety precautions are in place. Fortunately, all our boys and girls have increased their muscular strength, and not one has experienced an exercise-related injury. This is most likely due to the careful supervision that we provide to all our strength-training participants.

Others also recommend strength training for young people. Since 1985 several medical organizations, including the American Academy of Pediatrics, the American Orthopaedic Society for Sports Medicine, the Society of Pediatric Orthopaedics and the American College of Sports Medicine, have published guidelines for pre-adolescent strength training. These training guidelines were designed in conjunction with major fitness organizations, including the National Strength and Conditioning Association, the President's Council on Physical Fitness and Sports, the U.S. Olympic Committee, and the National Athletic Trainers Association. Now that's a pretty impressive list of supporters for youth strength training. The recently released United States Surgeon General's Report on Physical Activity and Health also stresses the need for boys and girls to participate regularly in physical activities that enhance muscle function. Furthermore, because muscular strength and power are required for success in most sports, it is likely that young athletes who strength train will perform better than those who do not strength train. What's more, strength training during childhood and adolescence may provide the foundation for dramatic gains in strength and power during adulthood.

Strength Training Versus Weightlifting

There is a difference between strength training and weightlifting. By definition, strength training is a planned and progressive means for exercising with appro-

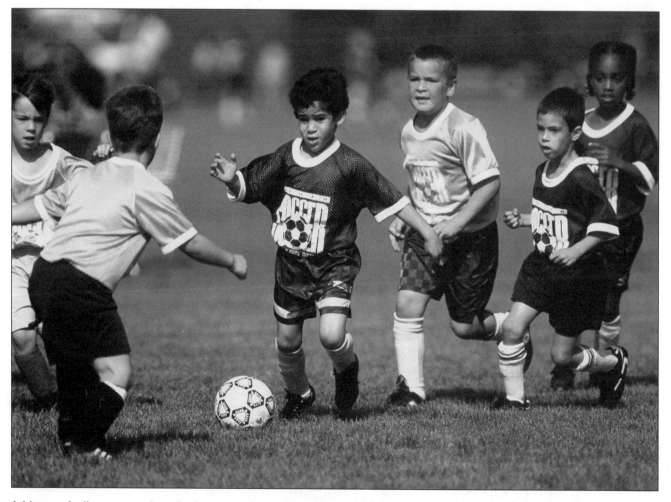

Athletes of all ages can benefit from muscle conditioning activities.

priate resistance, which you gradually increase as the musculoskeletal system becomes stronger. You can perform strength training with a variety of equipment, such as resistance machines, free weights (barbells and dumbbells), elastic bands, or body weight alone. Properly designed and supervised youth strength-training programs should be enjoyable activities in which every child gains strength and experiences success in a safe and supportive exercise environment.

Conversely, weightlifting is a sport in which participants typically work with heavy barbells and attempt to lift maximum weight loads in competitive events. Although well-coached weightlifting programs have their place, this book does not cover the competitive lifts, known as the clean and jerk, and the snatch. This book presents the principles and programs for sensible youth strength training, emphasizing the exercises and techniques that are fundamental for all youth, including young athletes.

Fundamental Fitness

There are two broad categories of youth, and both need strength training to attain a reasonable level of fundamental fitness. The larger category consists of those boys and girls who engage in little physical activity on a regular basis. Unlike children in earlier generations, they don't do many physical chores, don't play backyard sports, don't have many physical education classes, and don't engage in much vigorous activity. Instead, they spend most of their free time in passive pursuits such as watching television, playing video games, or surfing the Internet. These youth desperately need strength training to condition their muscles, tendons, ligaments, and bones. A fundamental level of musculoskeletal fitness is essential for youth to experience and enjoy a physically active lifestyle.

The other and much smaller category of young people consists of the sport participants. These are the kids who play soccer; do age-group swimming; take dance, gymnastics, and skating lessons; and participate in other organized sport activities. Although they get plenty of physical exercise, they also need a general program of strength training to ensure balanced muscle development and a low risk for overuse injuries. Basically, children should have good overall strength before engaging in competitive sports that can place excessive stress on an unconditioned musculo-skeletal system. An overemphasis on sport-specific skills typically provides too little stimulus for many major muscles and too much stress on other major muscles, with injury the likely result.

In the long term, sport participants who do not possess sufficient muscular strength are likely to drop out due to injury, failure, or frustration. This is why it is so important to develop fundamental fitness before

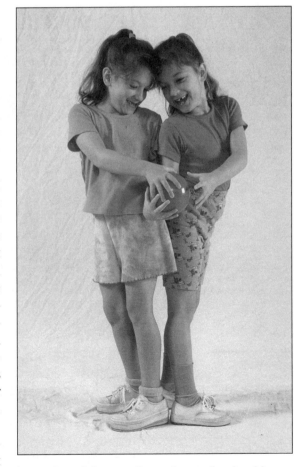

Strength training can be a fun and enjoyable activity for children.

specializing in skill training. According to the American College of Sports Medicine, children could prevent about 50 percent of overuse injuries in youth sports if they emphasized fundamental fitness more than sport-specific training. Also, when youngsters have well-conditioned muscles, they are more successful in mastering the motor skills required for high levels of sport performance.

With these things in mind, it should be obvious that strength training is a fundamental fitness activity for all boys and girls. In fact, strength training is a logical solution to the present problem of too many young people who are underactive and overweight. Youth who are strong and fit could reverse the present situation, in which most high school students do less than 60 minutes a week of vigorous physical activity and graduate with more hours in front of a television than in the classroom.

Strength-training programs provide sedentary students with positive after-school activity that enables them to enjoy purposeful exercise, experience personal improvement, and train cooperatively with friends in a supportive setting and exciting atmosphere. Because childhood is a critical period for developing lifelong attitudes and activity patterns, this is the best time to begin strength training. Research clearly indicates that participation in a supervised program of strength exercise can make a world of difference in a child's life.

Muscles, Bones, and Connective Tissue

The concept of fundamental fitness revolves around developing a strong and fit musculoskeletal system. The musculoskeletal system consists of the muscles, tendons, ligaments, and bones that enable us to move and perform physical activities. A strong musculoskeletal system prepares children for all types of physical activity and reduces the risk of sport-related injuries. Few things have as much positive impact on a young person's life as a well-conditioned musculoskeletal system.

You may have heard that children do not have sufficient levels of the muscle-building hormone testosterone to gain strength apart from normal growth and maturation. This is a false assumption. Although preadolescents and females of all ages have too little natural testosterone to develop large muscles, they can certainly increase their muscle strength. Boys and girls in research studies have improved their muscle strength as much as 74 percent in only two months of training. This is possible because strength development is associated with a variety of neuromuscular factors and does not solely depend on hormone levels.

Another misconception concerns growth retardation in children who train with weights. Nothing could be further from the truth. There has never been a report of stunted growth or reduced bone formation related to strength training. On the contrary, progressive strength exercise makes bones strong and resistant to injury. Because most of our bone mass is accrued during our youth years, this is the ideal time to enhance musculoskeletal strength and structure through properly designed resistance-training programs. Strength training may be beneficial for young girls to reduce their risk of osteoporosis later in life. Although strength training won't make children taller, it can contribute to physically developing their muscles, bones, tendons, and ligaments.

Getting Ready

Although there is no minimum age requirement for doing strength exercise, children should exhibit the emotional maturity to accept and follow directions before participating in a strength-training program. All participants should have a positive attitude toward the strength-training program. You should not force children to continue who do not look forward to their strength-training sessions. As a point of reference, boys and girls as young as age six have successfully completed youth strength-training programs.

Children who play organized sports (soccer, football, basketball, baseball, swimming, gymnastics, dance, skating, etc.) should also participate in some supervised strength-building activity. In fact, this should be standard procedure for young athletes to reduce their risk of injury, as well as to prepare them for more successful performance and satisfying participation in sports. Children should begin strength training at least two to three months before their sport season. Keep in mind that youth do not achieve athletic conditioning by playing sports but must get into shape *for* playing sports.

Although the concept of preseason conditioning for children may seem bizarre, it appears that many children who enter sports are unfit and ill prepared to handle the physical demands of practice and game situations. Therefore, it makes sense for aspiring young athletes to participate in a well-rounded fitness program before they begin sport-specific training. For over two generations, some parents and coaches have argued that early sport specialization was the key to later success in sports. However, it now appears that fitness conditioning and involvement in a variety of skills and activities relates more to later sport success than early sport specialization.

Under normal circumstances, it is not mandatory for apparently healthy children to have a medical examination before doing strength exercise. Of course, a physician should screen any child with known or suspected health problems, including illness or injury, before he or she participates in a strength-training program.

Due to age, size, and maturational differences, it is essential to address each child's needs and abilities in designing the strength-training program. That is, you should personalize the exercise protocol and training procedures as much as possible. Because an early-maturing youth has a strength advantage over a late-maturing child, take care to emphasize individual progress and to avoid weight-load comparisons. We advise that you address the reasons for program differences, as most children understand and appreciate the ability-based training approach.

Children who are active in organized sports may need to make some training adjustments before adding strength exercise to an already full schedule of physical pursuits. To prevent overtraining and permit appropriate recovery time, carefully evaluate the young athlete's weekly training. For example, a young gymnast should incorporate strength training into a redesigned workout schedule rather than simply adding it to the weekly training routine.

Perhaps the most important consideration for youth strength-training programs is that children are not merely miniature adults. Standard adult workout protocols may not be best for young people. For example, children respond better to high-repetition training (13 to 15) than to low-repetition training (6 to 8).

You must also clearly understand that strength programs practiced by college and professional athletes are unacceptable for boys and girls with immature bodies. Remember that children are less developed physically and psychologically, and they participate in strength training for different reasons than adult athletes. Basically, young strength trainers are motivated by learning new skills, making new friends, and having fun while exercising. Attempting to sell strength training to children on the basis that it can improve their quality of life is a losing proposition. Even though our society often highlights the importance of winning, remember that the major reason most young people engage in physical activity is to have fun. The focus of youth activity programs should be on positive experiences instead of stressful competition in which most children fail.

Acknowledging that there are some inherent risks in all physical endeavors, a properly designed and supervised strength-training program is a safe, purposeful, and productive activity for young people. In fact, with competent instruction and supervision, strength training is an ideal activity for most boys and girls, as it provides opportunity for progressive challenges and recurrent successes while building both physical prowess and self-confidence.

Summary

Despite preconceived concerns associated with youth strength training, medical and fitness organizations now promote strength training for children and adolescents, provided that they follow appropriate training guidelines. In addition to increasing the strength of muscles, bones, and connective tissue, regular participation in a strength-training program may better prepare young athletes for sport participation and may reduce the number and severity of sport-related injuries. With competent instruction and quality practice time, boys and girls can learn the skills needed for successful and enjoyable participation in strength-training activities.

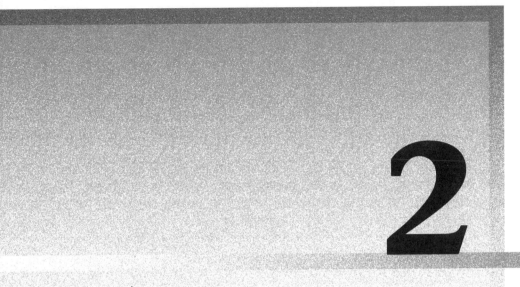

Program Prescriptions

With appropriate guidance young athletes can have fun while conditioning their muscles and developing a positive attitude about strength-training activities. The program we suggest allows both adolescent and preadolescent boys and girls the opportunity to work in a safe and stimulating environment through individually prescribed exercise methods.

You can strive for an injury-free program by introducing the many benefits of strength training and emphasizing the importance of proper exercise technique. Place high priority on education and motivation, which encourage the boys and girls to take a positive perspective and a sensible approach to their strength-training program. Of course, having competent instruction and close supervision is most helpful, and a low teacher-student ratio is important. Provide at least one instructor for every five participants. However, a ratio of one instructor for every 10 participants may be acceptable for experienced teenage exercisers.

Our basic advice for successful youth strength training is to design personalized programs that accommodate each child's physical abilities. Intense exercise sessions with short rest periods certainly have their place, but most children find such programs too demanding and discouraging. We believe it is better to underestimate participants' physical abilities and progress gradually to harder workouts and heavier weight loads than to do too much too soon and encounter setbacks or injuries.

We have regular and relevant conversations with the children, listening carefully to their concerns, as well as giving them plenty of encouragement, feedback, and positive reinforcement. On the other hand, we consistently and fairly enforce the training rules, foremost of which are no maximum lifting and no fast lifting. Our primary objectives are to help each child master his or her training system, use proper exercise technique, record workout information, and monitor personal progress.

Needless to say, we accept no form of horseplay in the exercise area. While our warm-up and cool-down components involve games and group activities such as aerobic dance, locomotor games, and relays, we do everything with order and control. If a child feels weak or fatigued, we adjust the training session accordingly. We make every effort to help the children feel competent, confident, and comfortable in the exercise environment.

Keep in mind that a safe exercise setting must be spacious, uncluttered, well ventilated, and well lighted. All training equipment should be in good working order and properly sized for the participants. Most children are too small for adult-sized weight machines, and adolescents may need an extra board or pad to fit into the machine properly. Of course, child-sized weight machines and free weights such as barbells and dumbbells are viable alternatives for small boys and girls. Be sure to provide adequate space around each exercise station and keep the floor clear of barbells, dumbbells, weight plates, and other materials. We insist that the youth dress appropriately for exercise, with supportive athletic shoes and clothing that permits freedom of movement.

Equipment Selection

With respect to strength equipment, we believe that sound training techniques and teaching methods are more important than the mode of exercise. For example, we have experienced excellent training effects from youth programs using free weights (barbells and dumbbells), and Nautilus machines (pushing and pulling exercises), as well as child-sized machines (weight stacks and plate loaded). We have also used rubber tubing, medicine balls, and body-weight exercises. All have proven safe and productive when children practice the prescribed training procedures. Although well-designed, single-station, child-sized machines have certain advantages, exercise technique is far more important than the type of exercise equipment used in training. The information in this book will enable youth to attain excellent strength development on all types of exercise equipment.

Although there are a variety of single-station machines, we suggest beginning with basic exercises for the major muscle groups, such as leg extensions, leg curls, leg presses, chest presses, seated rows, shoulder presses, biceps curls, and triceps pressdowns. We also emphasize midsection exercises for the typically under-developed lower-back and abdominal muscles. Trunk curls and trunk extensions performed with body weight or on appropriately sized machines work well for this purpose and thereby reduce the injury risk to this vulnerable area of the body.

Training Guidelines

Specific guidelines for safe, sensible, and successful youth strength-training programs have been identified. Several key exercise and medical associations, including the American Orthopaedic Society for Sports Medicine, the American Academy of Pediatrics, the American College of Sports Medicine, the Society of Pediatric Orthopaedics, the National Athletic Trainers Association, the U.S. Olympic Committee, the National Strength and Conditioning Association, and the President's Council on Physical Fitness and Sports, developed a collaborative position paper on strength training for preadolescent boys and girls. First presented in 1985, these youth strength-training guidelines provided the following directives.

Equipment

Children have used different types of strength-training equipment safely and effectively. Consider the following factors when evaluating youth-strength training equipment:

1. Equipment should be of appropriate design to accommodate the size and degree of maturity of the child or adolescent.
2. It should be cost-effective.
3. Equipment should be safe, free of defects, and inspected frequently.
4. It should be located in an uncrowded area free of obstructions with adequate lighting and ventilation.

Program Considerations

Children should genuinely appreciate the benefits and risks associated with youth strength training, and adults should have a solid understanding of strength-training principles. If you adhere to the following considerations, youth strength training has the potential to be a pleasurable and valuable experience.

1. The child must have the emotional maturity to accept coaching and instruction.
2. There must be adequate supervision by coaches who are knowledgeable about strength training and the special problems of prepubescents.
3. Strength training should be part of a comprehensive program to increase motor skills and fitness level.
4. The child should precede strength training by a warm-up period and follow it by a cool-down.
5. The program should emphasize dynamic concentric and ecocentric muscle actions.
6. The child should carry all exercises through a full range of motion.

Prescribed Program

Children should begin strength training at a level that is commensurate with their physical abilities and goals. While a variety of training programs have been developed for children, we recommend the following guidelines:

1. Strength training two or three times a week for 20- to 30-minute periods.
2. The child should apply no resistance until he or she can demonstrate proper form. Six to 15 repetitions equal one set; the child should do one to three sets per exercise.
3. Increase weight or resistance in one- to three-pound increments after the participant does 15 repetitions in good form.

These recommendations are just as relevant today as they were in 1985, but research studies conducted during the 1990s have enabled us to make a few refinements that enhance both the training efficiency and exercise effectiveness. For example, we have compared preadolescent strength gains achieved from fewer repetitions (6 to 8) with heavy weight loads and those attained from more repetitions (13 to 15) with moderate weight loads. Unlike adults, our findings indicate that preadolescent boys and girls do better with higher repetitions and moderate weight loads during the first few months of training. That is, children who train with weight loads that permit about 14 repetitions gain more strength than those who train with weight loads that permit about 7 repetitions.

Our studies suggest that preadolescents who perform one high-effort set of each exercise experience excellent strength gains. Therefore, single-set resistance training is an efficient and effective means for increasing muscle strength in young boys and girls. However, performing two or three sets per exercise may lead to even greater strength development over time, especially if done progressively. For example, we have attained our greatest strength gains using the DeLorme-Watkins training protocol, which requires a low-, moderate-, and high-effort set of each exercise. That is, the participant performs the first set with a light resistance for 10 repetitions, the second set with a moderate resistance for 10 repetitions, and the third set with a heavy resistance for 10 to 15 repetitions. When he or she can complete 15 repetitions, increase the resistance in all three sets slightly.

Although young people are prone to do things quickly, we insist on exercise control achieved through slow lifting and lowering movements. We generally require four to six seconds for each repetition, with two to three seconds each for the lifting and lowering movements. We believe that controlled movement speeds maximize strength development and minimize injury risk. Because fast movement speeds on weight machines involve momentum, they may reduce the exercise effect and training safety.

Our youth strength-training studies have shown similar results from two or three exercise sessions per week. On the one hand, most boys and girls like the strength-training program and are willing to exercise three days per week. On the other hand, two weekly workouts may make more sense for young people who are involved in additional physical activities such as dance, gymnastics, swimming, tennis, or team sports.

The training procedures for increasing muscle strength in boys and girls are simple and straightforward. Basically, youth should use enough resistance to complete between 10 and 15 repetitions at a controlled movement speed (four to six seconds per repetition). When they can complete15 repetitions in good form, increase the resistance by the smallest amount possible (typically one to three pounds). We recommend that children begin strength training with one set of each exercise, two or three days per week. Whenever possible, they should perform 8 to 10 strength exercises each training session.

The strength workout should include all the major muscle groups, which participants may accomplish by single- and multijoint exercise selections. Table 2.1 presents standard free-weight and machine exercises available on youth-sized equipment that address the major muscle groups.

All our exercisers begin with lightweight loads and progress gradually in small increments (typically two pounds). We permit a minute or two of rest between exercises until the youth increase their fitness level and familiarity with the training program. We also prefer to teach a few basic exercises and systematically add new exercises when the children are ready for more movements.

Once the boys and girls have mastered the fundamental training program, we may incorporate specialized exercises. Also, children may perform more sets of each exercise if desired. Of course, the key to advanced youth strength training is progressive participation in a well-designed and carefully supervised exercise program that leads to high levels of strength and increased interest in muscular fitness.

Program Design

All strength-training sessions should begin with a 10- to 15-minute warm-up period that includes low-intensity aerobic exercise and stretching. A proper warm-up prepares children and adolescents for strength-training activities and reduces the chance of a joint or muscle injury. Five to 10 minutes of aerobic exercise such as walking or calisthenics increases blood flow through active tissues and raises muscle and core temperature. We often incorporate lightweight (one- to two-pound) medicine ball exercises into the warm-up to stimulate the specific muscles and joints that the participants will use in the strength-training session.

Following the aerobic warm-up, participants should perform several stretching exercises for their upper and lower bodies. They should perform each stretch two or three times and hold it for at least 15 seconds. It is important to remind children to breathe normally while stretching and to reach a point where they feel a gentle pull, not pain. Remember that the warm-up period should not cause fatigue.

We recommend eight stretches for young strength trainers (see pages 15-18).

TABLE 2.1

Standard Free-Weight and Machine Exercises for the Major Muscle Groups

Muscle groups	Free-weight exercises	Machine exercises
Front thigh (quadriceps)	Dumbbell squat Dumbbell lunge Dumbbell step-up	Leg extension Leg press
Rear thigh (hamstrings)	Dumbbell squat Dumbbell lunge Dumbbell step-up	Leg curl Leg press
Inner thigh (hip adductors)	Dumbbell side lunge	Hip adduction
Outer thigh (hip abductors)	Dumbbell side lunge	Hip abduction
Lower leg (gastrocnemius and soleus)	Dumbbell heel raise	Heel raise
Chest (pectoralis major)	Dumbbell bench press	Chest press
Upper back (latissimus dorsi)	Dumbbell one-arm row Dumbbell pullover	Seated row Pullover Front pulldown
Shoulders (deltoids)	Dumbbell lateral raise	Overhead press
Front arms (biceps)	Dumbbell biceps curl Dumbbell incline biceps curl	Biceps curl
Rear arms (triceps)	Dumbbell triceps kickback Dumbbell triceps overhead extension	Triceps extension
Lower back (erector spinae)	Prone back raise	Low-back extension
Abdominals (rectus abdominis)	Trunk curl	Abdominal curl
Forearms (extensors and flexors)	Wrist roller Dumbbell wrist extension Dumbbell wrist curl	Super forearm

CHEST STRETCH

Interlock your fingers behind your head and gently move your elbows backward.

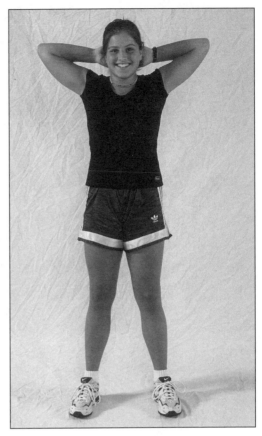

TRICEPS AND LAT STRETCH

Reach one arm behind your head as if you were trying to scratch your back. Gently pull the elbow toward the midline of your body. Repeat on the other side.

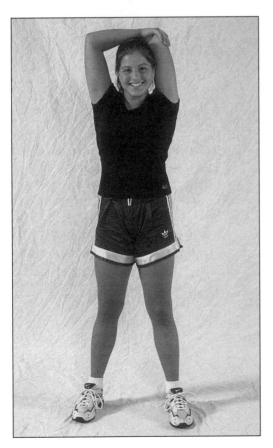

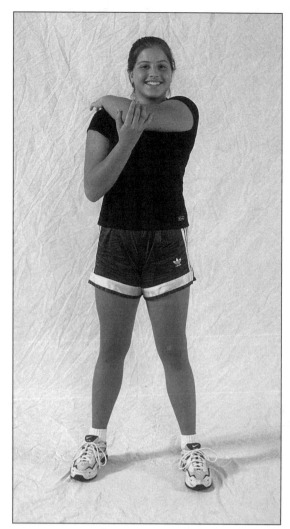

UPPER-BACK STRETCH

Reach across your body with one arm and place the hand on the opposite shoulder. Gently press the elbow across your body. Repeat on the other side.

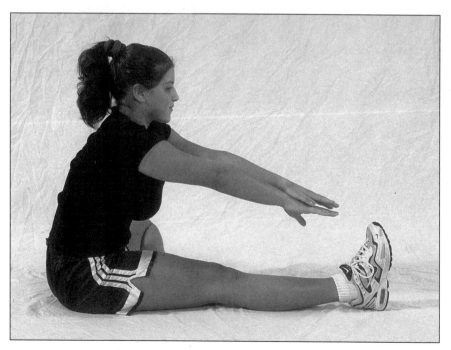

HAMSTRING STRETCH

Sit upright with one leg straight in front of your body and the other knee bent with the heel against the inner thigh of the extended leg. Bend at the hip and gently lean forward while keeping the extended leg straight. Repeat on the other side.

LOW-BACK AND HIP STRETCH

Sit upright on the floor with both legs straight in front of your body. Cross one leg over the other and place the opposite arm against the bent knee to assist with torso rotation. Repeat on the other side.

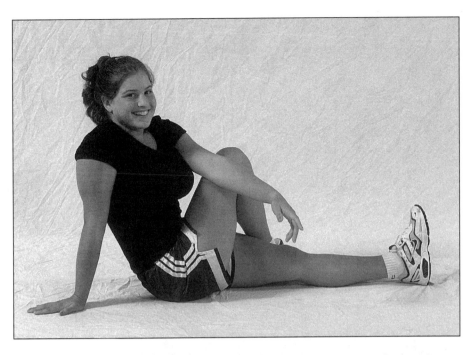

INNER-THIGH STRETCH

Sit upright with your knees bent and the soles of your feet touching. Grasp your ankles and gently press your elbows against your knees.

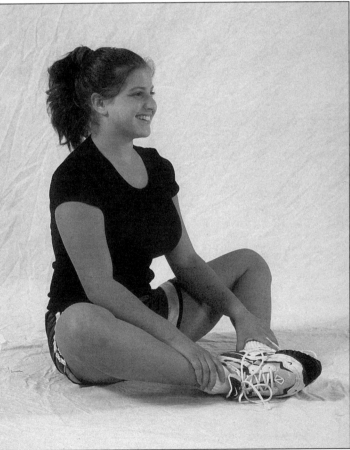

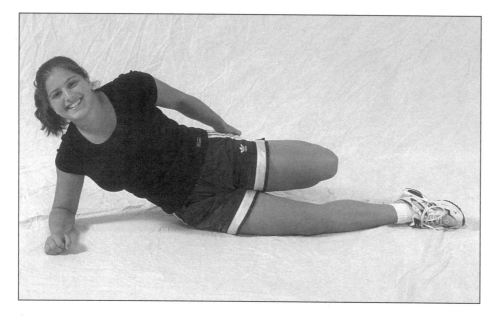

QUADRICEPS STRETCH

Lie on your side and bend one knee toward your buttocks. Grasp the ankle with one hand and gently pull your heel toward your buttocks. Repeat on the other side.

CALF STRETCH

With your arms extended in front of your body, place both hands against a wall for support. Bend the knee of the front leg and keep the back leg straight with the heel on the floor. Repeat on the other side.

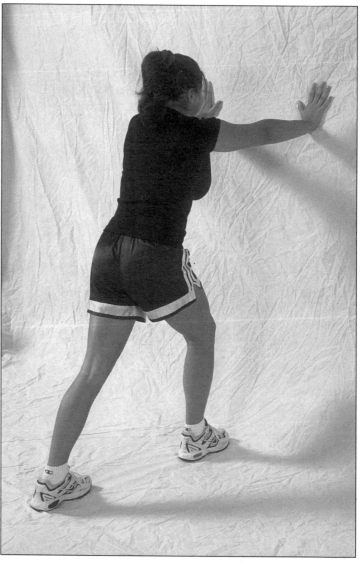

We put as much effort into promoting positive attitudes as we do on the physical aspects of the strength-training program. We promote gradual improvement and continually remind the students that it takes time to develop strength and master new skills. We also stress the training consistency and reward the children for regular participation. We keep track of attendance on a large poster board that we display in our youth fitness center. We ask children who regularly come to class to assist with exercise demonstrations, and teenagers who have graduated from our program sometimes return to provide encouragement and instruction. We give rewards such as water bottles, Frisbees, and T-shirts for consistent participation. We often treat the class to heart-healthy snacks, and at the end of each program all participants receive a certificate of completion signed by the course instructors (see figure 2.1). Throughout the program we take the time to acknowledge birthdays, graduations, and other special events.

To avoid a winners and losers atmosphere in the weight room, we emphasize intrinsic factors and individual achievement without comparing weight loads or performance abilities. For example, we use personal workout logs so the children record their own training efforts and focus on personal improvement (see figure 2.2). We encourage each participant to ask questions, and we interact as

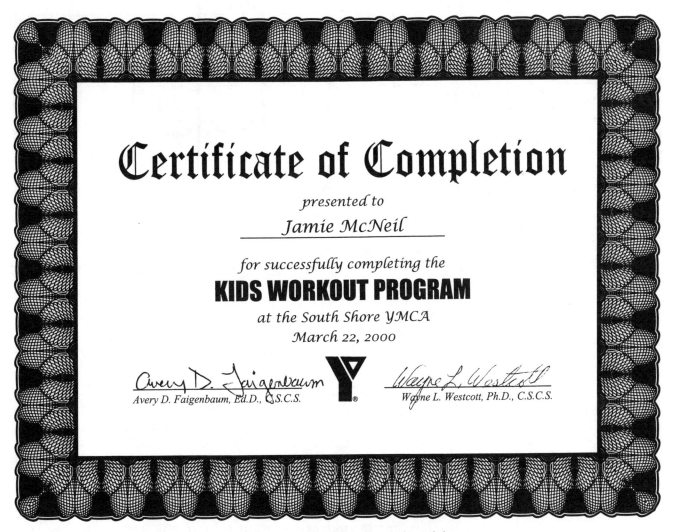

Figure 2.1 Children like to receive certificates of completion for their training.

Kids Workout Log

Name: _Sue Ramsden_   **Age:** _9_   **Class:** _M, W 3:15 pm_

Comments: _Allergic to Nuts_   **Telephone:** _479-8500_

Exercise:	Seat Position:	Date: 3/20 Wt: / Reps:	Date: 3/22 Wt: / Reps:	Date: Wt: / Reps:	Date: Wt: / Reps:	Date: Wt: / Reps:	Date: Wt: / Reps:	Date: Wt: / Reps:
(1) DB SQUAT		8 / 10	8 / 11					
(2) LEG CURL	2	10 / 10	10 / 11					
(3) DB HEEL RAISE		10 / 10	10 / 11					
(4) CHEST PRESS	2	20 / 10	20 / 11					
(5) SEATED ROW	1	15 / 10	15 / 11					
(6) DB LATERAL RAISE		3 / 10	3 / 11					
(7) DB BICEPS CURL		5 / 10	5 / 11					
(8) TRICEPS PRESSDOWN		10 / 10	10 / 11					
(9) PRONE BACK RAISE		Reps: 10	Reps: 11	Reps:	Reps:	Reps:	Reps:	Reps:
(10) TRUNK CURL		Reps: 10	Reps: 11	Reps:	Reps:	Reps:	Reps:	Reps:

Figure 2.2 Training logs are an effective way to track individual improvement.

much as possible with every boy and girl. We sometimes stop an exercise to correct technique or reduce the resistance if the child is not performing it properly. However, we do our best to make all recommendations in a positive and friendly manner, working together to attain our training objectives.

Summary

The prescribed strength-training program for children and adolescents should include a variety of exercises that address the major muscle groups of the body. Children and adolescents can safely use different types of equipment, including weight machines and free weights, provided that qualified supervision is present and participants understand the importance of proper exercise technique. Parents and coaches need to address individual needs and concerns and should fairly enforce training rules for the safety of all participants. Don't overlook the importance of having fun and developing a positive attitude toward strength-training activities. With appropriate guidance and supervision, children and adolescents can learn to embrace self-improvement and feel good about their accomplishments.

Correct Technique and
Injury Prevention

Strength training can be a safe and effective way to condition the musculo-skeletal system if the program is followed appropriately and within guide-lines. Over the past 15 years, we have worked with children ages 8 to 16 who have enjoyed participating in our youth strength-training programs. Recently we have even introduced children as young as six to the benefits of training. Despite preconceived concerns, research studies strongly indicate that supervised youth strength-training programs have a lower injury risk than other sports and activities in which children regularly participate. In fact, it seems that the forces children place on their musculoskeletal systems when participating in strength training are likely to be less in duration and magnitude of exposure than what they would generate participating in soccer, football, or gymnastics.

Although adults and children who strength train may have similar goals, the focus of youth strength-training programs should be on intrinsic factors such as skill improvement, personal successes, and having fun. We place a high value on participation and positively reinforce children who actively participate in the

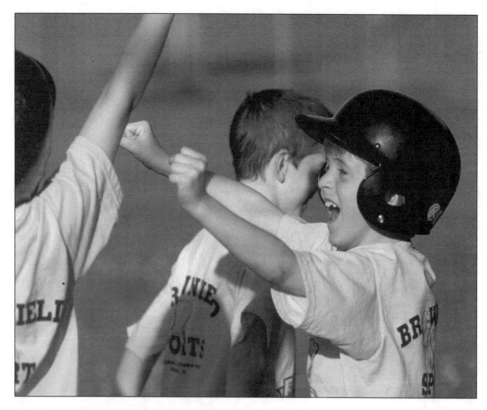

Physical activities can be both fun and rewarding.

workouts. Adults need to realize that the slogan "No pain, no gain" does not apply when working with boys and girls, most of whom have never experienced strength exercise before. Most adults and children enjoy physical activity if it is appropriately prescribed. Yet we are troubled by the increasing number of participants who drop out because the exercise program was too intense, too time consuming, or simply not fun. Parents, teachers, and coaches need to understand the uniqueness of children and the importance of adhering to safety concerns. The focus of our program is not on the amount of weight that children can lift, but on developing proper form and technique for a variety of strength-building exercises. Our goal is to teach children how to strength train properly so they can continue this important exercise for a lifetime.

To ensure the safety of your youth strength-training program, you need to take the following steps:

- Parents must complete a health history questionnaire on each child. If there is evidence of a preexisting medical concern, they must obtain physician approval before the child begins the program.
- Instructors must make sure the exercise area is adequately ventilated and free of clutter.
- Children should wear comfortable attire that does not restrict movement patterns and athletic footwear that provides good traction and prevents slipping.
- Children must not wear necklaces of any type, including those that hold keys, when strength training.
- Children should not chew gum during class.
- Children should drink water before, during, and after class.
- Instructors must begin the training with light weights to allow appropriate adjustments and gradual progression.
- Children must focus on proper exercise technique rather than the amount of weight they lift.
- Instructors who are knowledgeable in strength training must supervise every class.

Understanding Children

It is most important that knowledgeable adults who understand and appreciate the physical and psychological characteristics of children teach them how to strength train. Unlike adults, children are still growing and are therefore more prone to certain types of injury. For example, children may damage growth cartilage located at the end of long bones, near the tendon insertion and on the joint surface, if the forces on them are too great. Damage to the growth cartilage is a serious concern because it can stop the bone from growing. Although injuries to the growth cartilage have been reported in children who trained with weights, these injuries typically happened when children attempted to press near-maximum weights overhead in an unsupervised environment. Fortunately, this type of injury has not been reported in any youth strength-training program that incorporated an appropriate progression of training loads and close supervision. To minimize the chance of injury to the growth cartilage, children should not perform overhead lifts with near-maximum resistance, and they should always follow proper and progressive training procedures. Children should learn how to perform overhead lifts with a broomstick handle or a piece of PVC piping, emphasizing proper form and technique.

Damage to the growth cartilage can also occur if children repeatedly participate in sports and recreational activities without giving their bodies a chance to recover. The problem is that repetitive stress to the growing area of the bone results in microtraumas, which need time to heal and recover. Without adequate recovery, the microtraumas eventually result in what is commonly known as an overuse injury. Although strength training reduces the incidence of overuse injuries in youth sport participants, it is important for parents and coaches to consider the total exercise picture before adding strength training to a child's sport program. Just like other physical activities, strength training contributes to the overall repetitive stress on the young musculoskeletal system, and therefore the child must sensibly incorporate it into his or her activity program.

If you incorporate strength training without considering other activities, the overall stress on the growing child may be too great, and the child may experience an overuse injury. We believe that you should design strength training into a year-round conditioning program that changes periodically. During this time children can improve their overall fitness levels, and you can identify and correct any specific needs, such as muscle imbalances. In some cases, children may need to decrease the time they spend practicing sport-specific skills to allow time for preparatory conditioning. Further, we must realize that children with immature musculoskeletal systems may not be able to tolerate the same amount of exercise that some of their friends can withstand. Thus we always treat each child as an individual, and pay close attention to his or her response to the strength-training program.

Being a Teacher

Adults must have a thorough understanding of youth strength-training guidelines and should speak with children at a level they understand. Clearly explain instructions to all children and demonstrate exercises properly. Because children

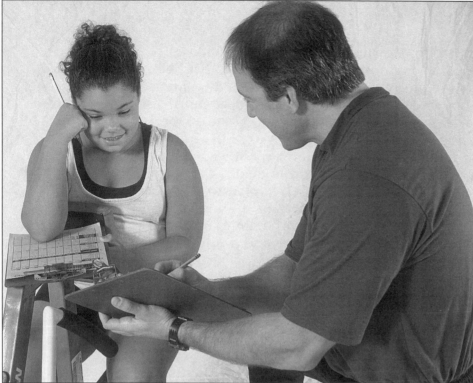

Teach children how to record their workout on a training log.

tend to listen with their eyes, we make a point to demonstrate every exercise to all the children. We often have experienced boys and girls demonstrate the exercises for the class. We continually provide feedback to the children and are sensitive that most of them have never trained with weights before. It is important to be patient with children and allow them the opportunity to master the performance of an exercise before moving to more advanced training techniques.

We begin our youth strength-training programs with a major focus on education. We do not lecture to children in a classroom, but we do spend time in the exercise room showing children how to strength train safely. We discuss the value of physical activity and introduce the children to proper exercise technique, training guidelines, and safety procedures. Most notably, we focus on the technique of each exercise rather than the amount of weight lifted. During the first few training sessions, we develop the concept of a fitness workout that includes warm-up exercises, stretches, and a cool-down period. We carefully monitor the children's tolerance of the exercise session, and we remind them that it takes time to learn new skills and attain high levels of strength fitness.

Adults also need to look beyond the mere prescription of sets and repetitions when working with children. Do not limit the goal of the program to increasing muscular strength, but include teaching children about their bodies, promoting lifetime fitness, and generating positive attitudes toward strength training and exercise in general. Above all, children need to enjoy the experience of strength training and have fun during their workouts. We teach children how to use training logs so they can record each exercise set and keep track of personal progress.

Over the years, hundreds of children have participated in our youth strength-training classes. Although we are confident that the boys and girls have successfully learned new physical skills, no child has ever said, "Thanks Coach, my blood pressure dropped 10 points and my bones are stronger than ever." Children want to be active like adults, but for different reasons. Most children want to participate in activities with friends, experience something new and challenging, and have fun.

Using Equipment Safely

You need to carefully evaluate the equipment used in the youth strength-training program. Although children can effectively use all sorts of equipment, from medicine balls to weight machines, they should always follow safety precautions. If we use weight machines, we make sure each child properly fits into each machine. Due to differences in body size and shape, it is often necessary to make a few adjustments by adding a pad or changing the position of the resistance lever. As each child grows, you may need to make equipment modifications accordingly. It is also important to place the weight machines far enough apart to allow easy access and maneuverability. If children strength train at home, parents need to find safe places to store the weights so younger brothers and sisters don't get hurt playing with them.

Parents, teachers, and coaches should take the time before every class to ensure that the exercise room is safe and free of clutter. Barbells and dumbbells should be placed on the appropriate racks and the location of the weight machines should allow for easy access. Overcrowded and poorly designed exercise rooms with too many pieces of equipment increase the likelihood that a child may bump into the equipment or walk into the end of a barbell. Properly designed exercise areas are not only more efficient places to train, but they are also safer. In addition to developing age-appropriate workouts for young weight trainers, we always design our youth strength-training areas with safety in mind.

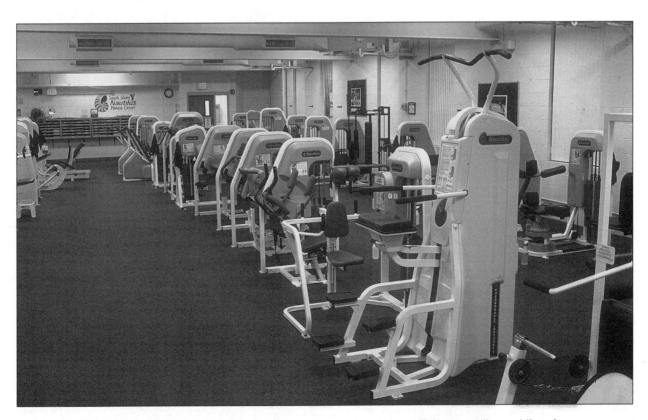

Training facilities should be designed for exercise safety and training efficiency while enabling free movement around resistance equipment.

We are aware of the exploratory nature of children and therefore remove or disassemble any potential hazards or broken equipment from the exercise room before classes begin. If children use dumbbells or barbells, we always start with a light weight so they have an opportunity to develop the balance and coordination necessary to perform the exercise correctly. Always teach proper spotting procedures to teenagers who want to perform free-weight exercises, such as the squat and the bench press. When using dumbbells and barbells, a spotter can help return the weight to the starting position if the child cannot complete the last repetition. If children under the age of 12 perform free-weight exercises that require a spotter, we suggest that an adult provide the necessary assistance.

Keeping It Progressive

The strength-training program designed for each child should be commensurate with his or her individual abilities. We recognize that children will get stronger at different rates and therefore encourage them to progress at their own pace so they can experience success without getting hurt. Too often the initial program is overly intense for beginners, and the child's developing musculoskeletal system may be ill prepared to handle the stress of such a program. It is important to begin strength training with light loads so children have an opportunity to develop proper form and technique on each exercise.

To keep the program fresh and challenging, increase the weights gradually as children are able to perform the desired number of repetitions with the correct form and technique. However, a one- to three-pound increase in weight is often consistent with a 5- to 10-percent increase in overload. That is to say, if a child performed 12 repetitions with 10 pounds on a biceps curl exercise, he or she should increase the weight to 11 pounds and decrease repetitions to 8. Although adults may increase their weights by 5 to 10 pounds at a time, this is too much for children who typically use much lighter weights than adults. We also challenge the students by adding new exercises that require a higher degree of skill, yet are attainable with practice.

Summary

With appropriate guidance and instruction, strength training can become a healthy habit that lasts a lifetime. The key is to understand the uniqueness of children and appreciate the fact that most children participate in physical activities to learn something new, make friends, and have fun. Take the time to teach children the proper form and technique on each exercise and be sure to answer any questions they may have. Encourage children to master the performance of basic exercises so they can progress to advanced training techniques. Throughout the program, evaluate each child's responses to the training program and recognize that children will get stronger at different rates. Keeping the fun in fitness will spark an interest in lifelong physical activity.

4

Eating for Strength

Now that you are ready to begin a youth strength-training program, you may have some questions about proper nutrition and daily dietary requirements. For example, you may have heard that strength training increases the need for protein, calcium, and other nutrients found in muscles and bones. Although this may be true to some degree, it is neither necessary nor desirable to follow specialized diets or spend lots of money on food supplements. Generally, home-cooked meals including a variety of grains, vegetables, fruits, and low-fat meat and dairy products are best from a nutritional perspective. Unfortunately, as society has become faster-paced, home-cooked meals have become less common, and supermarket shelves have become well stocked with high-fat, high-sugar, and high-salt foods. It is not surprising that one problem many youth may experience is weak nutrition.

Weak nutrition may be defined as meals and snacks that are too high in fat and too low in essential nutrients. The essential nutrients include protein (amino acids), calcium, potassium, minerals, and vitamins, as well as carbohydrates for energy and water for all body functions.

In recent years, particularly among teenagers, young adults, and athletes, power eating has become popular. This nutritional discipline restricts fat to about 20 to 25 percent of daily calories, increases nutrient-dense carbohydrates to about 55 to

60 percent of daily calories, and includes about 20 percent protein calories for building muscle tissue. Before adding protein for bigger muscles, however, it is important to keep in mind that muscle is over 75 percent water. Without question, the most important component of power eating is water, and active youth should drink at least eight glasses of water (or healthy alternatives such as fruit juices or low-fat milk) every day. It is also important to keep in mind that consuming excess amounts of protein in an attempt to alter a child's muscle development will not serve its purpose and may put the child at risk of health problems.

Children's Nutritional Needs

The Food Guide Pyramid developed by the United States Department of Agriculture models a strong nutrition program for children. As illustrated in figure 4.1, the Food Guide Pyramid includes several daily servings from the grain, vegetable, and fruit groups to ensure ample energy, as well as essential vitamins and minerals. It recommends fewer servings of low-fat meat and milk products to provide muscle-building proteins and bone-building calcium. The top of the Food Guide Pyramid is sparse servings of fat foods, primarily in the form of oils or sweets.

Although the Food Guide Pyramid presents a healthy and powerful eating pattern, many youth follow a completely opposite nutritional lifestyle. It is not unusual for teens and preteens to eat far more candy bars, corn chips, french fries, cheeseburgers, and ice cream (all of which are 50 to 80 percent fat) than apples, oranges, bananas, salads, cooked vegetables, rice, whole grains, fish, chicken, low-fat milk, and yogurt. Of course, the latter foods are low in fat and high in nutrients, making them much better selections. However, motivating a youth to *want* the healthier food selections is a key to developing a healthier lifestyle for the child. You can do this in the following ways.

First, encourage healthy eating patterns early. While the child is young, teach him or her to enjoy trying new fruits such as seedless clementines or papaya. If a child sees an adult eating something new, and if it looks good, he or she is naturally curious. To go one step further, when a child sees something new and does not have the alternate choice of a high-fat snack, he or she will naturally opt for what is available.

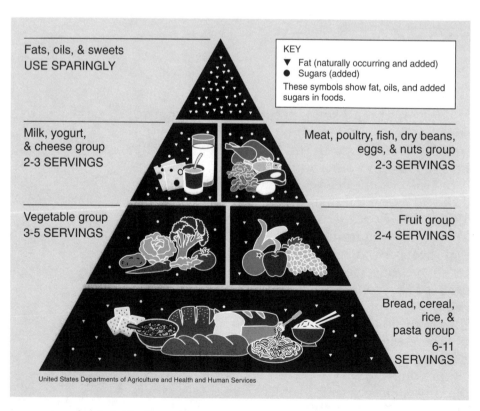

Figure 4.1 Food Guide Pyramid.

Another idea is to make certain snacks a tradition. For families, if Friday night is family time, be sure to have staples on hand such as raw baby carrots and fat-free ranch dressing. Carrots are naturally sweet and children love them. Another popular idea is sliced apples with cinnamon and sugar. Combine cinnamon and sugar in a small shaker for quick and easy preparation.

Role modeling plays an important part in developing healthy eating habits in children. Even as adults tend to eat those snacks most readily available in the household, during fitness programs, or at other social events, so the children will follow suit. If a child sees an adult consuming a bag of potato chips, his or her hand is going to reach for the same thing. If an adult routinely enjoys high sugar or high fat snacks how can he or she say no when the child asks for the same? This doesn't mean you have to sacrifice sweets completely. When choosing store-bought snacks, opt for the ones that are low in fat. Entenmann's offers some good choices; Sunshine is noted for their healthy products; SnackWells, Healthy Choice, Sweet Escapes, and Weight Watchers also have some appealing low-fat options.

This is not to say children (and adults) should not enjoy occasional pizzas or cookies with milk, but you should balance foods high in fat with several selections from the vegetable, fruit, and grain categories daily. As mentioned earlier in this chapter, we do not recommend additional protein foods or supplements to accelerate muscle development.

Protein Requirements

Taking too much protein is problematic for several reasons. First, the body does not use extra protein if sufficient protein is available. With few exceptions, boys and girls eat more than enough protein foods to satisfy all their muscle-building requirements. The body simply puts the excess protein into storage after the liver converts it to fat.

Unlike carbohydrates and fats, protein contains a waste component (nitrogen) that the body must neutralize and excrete. This chemical conversion uses calcium for the neutralization process, which may decrease body stores of this important mineral. Also, high protein concentrations make the kidneys work hard in the excretion process.

For these reasons, additional protein intake offers no muscle-building advantage for children or adults. How much protein is necessary for youth who participate in strength-training programs? Generally, one gram of protein for every two pounds of body weight is sufficient for meeting the metabolic needs and muscle-building requirements of teens and preteens.

For example, a boy or girl who weighs 100 pounds should eat approximately 50 grams of protein a day for optimum physical function. Because one ounce of meat (e.g., fish, chicken, turkey, lean beef) provides about seven grams of protein, an eight-ounce serving of meat should fulfill the daily protein requirement. Likewise, one cup of low-fat dairy products (e.g., milk, yogurt, cottage cheese) provides about eight grams of protein. Therefore, three servings of low-fat dairy foods provide about half the daily need for protein. Because most youth typically consume at least this much meat and milk, as well as other protein-containing foods daily, their muscles should be well supplied with protein and highly responsive to strength exercise.

Vitamins and Minerals

Many people believe that we do not obtain enough vitamins and minerals in our daily meals. However, this is only true if we do not eat a variety of foods as recommended in the Food Guide Pyramid. Youth and adults who consume several daily servings of grains, vegetables, and fruit, and a few servings of meat and milk should not lack any essential vitamins or minerals.

Of course, children who do not eat regular or varied meals may risk vitamin or mineral deficiency. Although we can easily remedy this problem by taking daily vitamin and mineral supplements, it is preferable to obtain our nutrients from the foods we eat. In addition to providing proteins, carbohydrates, fats, vitamins, and minerals, foods supply bulk and fiber necessary for desirable digestion and elimination.

Recently there has been considerable emphasis on antioxidant vitamins, especially vitamins A, C, and E. Fortunately, it is not difficult to attain plenty of these vitamins through healthy eating habits. For example, vitamin C is prevalent in citrus fruits and juices, tomatoes, potatoes, peppers, strawberries, melons, and many other fruits and vegetables. Vitamin A is found in most orange foods, such as cantaloupe, carrots, squash, sweet potatoes, and apricots. The best sources of vitamin E are wheat germ and fish, but you can also obtain it from sweet potatoes, almonds, and sunflower seeds.

Carbohydrates

Eating appropriate energy-releasing foods before and after strength workouts can enhance the training effort and recovery processes. Carbohydrates are the real power foods that serve as the primary energy source for strength exercise. Although all carbohydrates (grains, fruits, and vegetables) supply fuel for physical activity, some release energy slowly and others release energy quickly. Carbohydrates that break down slowly have a low glycemic index, and we recommend them before working out because they provide sustained energy and staying power. Carbohydrates that break down quickly have a high glycemic index because they enter the bloodstream fast and are effective for rapidly replenishing energy stores after exercising.

Before training eat foods that have a *low* glycemic index, including carrots, apples, pears, chocolate milk, low-fat fruit yogurt, dried apricots, bananas, and whole milk.

After training eat foods that have a *high* glycemic index, including Gatorade, cornflakes, rice cakes, vanilla wafers, graham crackers, honey, bagels, and raisins.

Snack Foods

We often ask children to avoid snacks between meals so they will have a good appetite for healthful food selections at breakfast, lunch, and dinner. Although this is good advice, active boys and girls may benefit from midmorning and midafternoon snacks. These energy-replacement selections should be small, nutritious, and accompanied with fluids.

Here are some healthy snacking ideas children may enjoy:

- Apple juice, orange juice, grape juice, or vegetable juice
- Banana and milk
- Raisins and milk
- Sliced apples with sugar and cinnamon
- Sliced apples with a thin layer of peanut butter
- Carrot sticks with nonfat ranch dressing
- Low-fat yogurt or cottage cheese
- Seedless grapes or clementines

Children who have a sweet tooth may want to substitute dried fruit (e.g., raisins, dates, figs, prunes, apricots) for candy and pastry. However dried fruit provides similar sweetness but contains almost no fat, making it a much healthier snack food than candy and pastry. Children who prefer high-sugar cereals may enjoy honey nut varieties. Honey Nut Shredded Wheat cereal makes a good whole-wheat snack.

Youth who like to munch on chips may substitute unsalted nuts or seeds (e.g., almonds, pecans, cashews, peanuts, sunflower seeds) as crunchy alternatives. Although nuts and seeds are high in oils, they contain many valuable nutrients and are healthier than foods high in saturated fats.

Basics for Healthy Eating

The Food Guide Pyramid presented in figure 4.1 provides guidelines for healthy eating that apply to adults and youth. Because small children need less food, they should eat fewer servings than adults in each category, but maintain the same relative proportions. That is, they should go heavy on grains, vegetables, and fruit; moderate on lean meats and low-fat dairy products; and light on fats, oils, and sweets. Let's consider each food category more carefully.

Grains

Grains include all kinds of foods made from wheat, oats, corn, rice, barley, and the like. Examples of grain foods include cereals, breads, pasta, pancakes, rice cakes, tortillas, bagels, muffins, corn bread, rice pudding, and chocolate cake. Obviously, some grain-based foods such as cakes, cookies, and pastries contain a lot of fat, and you should eat them sparingly. As mentioned, low-fat variations of these foods are available in local supermarkets.

All grains are high in carbohydrates, and some grains or parts of grains, such as wheat germ, are also good sources of protein. Whole grains are typically rich in vitamins B6, A, and E, as well as minerals such as zinc, copper, and iron. Whole grains are also good sources of soluble and insoluble fiber. Studies have shown that soluble fiber may help reduce blood cholesterol levels. Insoluble fiber helps with bowel regularity and may prevent gastrointestinal disorders. To determine whether a product contains whole grains, simply refer to the ingredient list. The first item should be labeled "whole" or "whole grain," such as whole wheat, whole corn, or whole rice.

The Food Guide Pyramid recommends 6 to 11 servings of grains every day. A serving is equivalent to a slice of bread or one-half cup of cooked pasta, so achieving the 6 to 11 servings is not difficult.

Vegetables

Like grains, vegetables are excellent sources of carbohydrates, vitamins, and fiber. Vegetables come in all sizes, shapes, colors, and nutritional characteristics, and they are low in calories. Orange vegetables are typically good sources of vitamin A and beta-carotene. This category includes carrots, sweet potatoes, and winter squash. Green vegetables are characteristically high in vitamins B2 and folic acid. Some green vegetables are peas, beans, broccoli, asparagus, spinach, and lettuce. A light vinaigrette salad dressing accompanying any of these vegetables may be more tasty for a child. Red vegetables provide ample amounts of vitamin C. The best known vegetables in this category are tomatoes and red peppers. Other vegetables are essentially white, at least under the skin. These include cauliflower, summer squash, potatoes, and radishes, many of which are good sources of vitamin C.

The Food Guide Pyramid recommends three to five daily servings of vegetables. One serving is one-half cup of any raw vegetable, except lettuce and sprouts, which require one cup per serving. Because heating reduces water content, cooked vegetables require less space than uncooked vegetables and serving sizes may be smaller. Likewise, vegetable juices are more concentrated and require only one-half cup per serving.

It is a good idea to eat some vegetables raw and to steam or microwave other vegetables for nutrient retention. In addition, fresh and frozen vegetables have more nutritional value and are lower in sodium than canned vegetables.

Fruit

Fruit is the counterpart to vegetables, low in calories, with as much variety and nutritional value. All fruit choices are high in carbohydrates and vitamins, and many provide excellent sources of fiber. A fruit's color often indicates the type of vitamin present.

As you probably know, citrus fruits, such as oranges, grapefruit, and lemons, are loaded with vitamin C. Like orange-colored vegetables, orange-colored fruit, including cantaloupe, apricots, and papaya, are rich in vitamin A and beta-carotene. Both green fruit, such as honeydew melon and kiwi, and red fruit, such as strawberries and cherries, are high in vitamin C. Yellow fruit includes peaches, mangos, and pineapples, all of which are good sources of vitamin C. Fruit that is white, at least on the inside, includes apples, pears, and bananas, all of which are high in potassium.

Dried fruits are nutrient dense, and the natural sweetness makes them healthy substitutes for high-fat snacks such as candy bars. Raisins, dates, figs, and prunes are all superb energy sources, and prunes are the single best source of dietary fiber.

TABLE 4.1

Fruit—One Serving Size

2 tbsp raisins	1 pear	1/4 papaya
3 dates	3 apricots	1/2 mango
3 prunes	1/2 grapefruit	5 kumquats
1/2 c grapes	3/4 c pineapple	1 c honeydew
1 apple	2 kiwi	1 1/4 c strawberries
1 banana	1/2 pomegranate	1 1/4 c watermelon
1 peach	1/4 cantaloupe	

The Food Guide Pyramid recommends two to four servings of fruit every day. Table 4.1 presents examples of a variety of fruits in one serving portions. You will notice that one serving varies considerably, depending on the type of fruit you eat. For example, it takes one-quarter of a melon or one-half of a grapefruit to equal three dates or two tablespoons of raisins. The difference is water content. Fresh fruit contains lots of water, whereas dried fruit is a high-density carbohydrate. If you prefer your fruit in liquid form, one-half cup of fruit juice equals one serving, but has less fiber than whole fruit.

Milk Products

The Food Guide Pyramid recommends two to three daily servings of low-fat dairy products, including milk, yogurt, and cheese. These foods are excellent sources of protein and calcium. Because whole milk products are high in fat, you should be selective at the dairy counter. For example, one-percent milk, low-fat yogurt, and nonfat cottage cheese offer heart-healthy alternatives to high-fat dairy selections.

One-quarter cup of low-fat cottage cheese has similar nutritional value to one cup of one-percent milk. Although there are many sources of dietary protein, children may have difficulty obtaining sufficient calcium unless they regularly consume milk products. If your child has problems digesting milk (lactose intolerance), try to regularly provide other foods that are high in calcium, such as tofu, leafy greens, beans, broccoli, and sesame seeds.

Meats

According to the Food Guide Pyramid, this category includes meat, poultry, fish, eggs, nuts, and dry beans. All these foods are good sources of protein, although some also contain significant amounts of fat. Table 4.2 presents sample foods in the meat category according to their fat content. You will note that how you prepare the meat has a lot do to with how much fat it contains.

Although there are differences in fat content, the amount of protein found in one serving is consistent throughout the various types of meat. As you can see

TABLE 4.2

Fat Content of Meat

Low fat	Medium fat	High fat
All fish	Chicken with skin	Beef ribs
Egg whites	Turkey with skin	Pork ribs
Chicken without skin	Roast beef	Corned beef
Turkey without skin	Roast pork	Sausage
Venison	Roast lamb	Lunch meat
Rabbit	Veal cutlet	Ground pork
Top round	Ground beef	Hot dogs
Eye of round	Steaks	Fried chicken
Sirloin	Canned salmon	Fried fish
Flank steak	Oil-packed tuna	Nuts
Veal	Whole eggs	Peanuts
Dry beans	Pork chops	Peanut butter

TABLE 4.3

Meat—One Serving Size

3 oz fish	1 tbsp peanut butter
3 oz poultry	1/4 c cooked dry beans
3 oz meat (beef, poultry, lamb, etc.)	1/4 c tuna
1 egg or 2 egg whites	1/4 c tofu

from table 4.3, three ounces of meat, poultry, and fish (about the size of a deck of cards) have the same amount of protein as do one-quarter cup of cooked dry beans and one-quarter cup of tuna. Children should consume two to three servings, for a total of six to nine ounces, from meat groups daily.

Fats

The smallest section of the Food Guide Pyramid is the fat group, which we should consume sparingly. Although all fats contain more than nine calories per gram, some fats are more desirable than others from a health perspective. For example, consuming saturated fats (such as those found in mayonnaise, butter, and sour cream) puts an individual at higher risk for developing heart disease than eating monounsaturated fats (such as those found in olive oil and canola oil) and polyunsaturated fats (such as those found in corn oil). See table 4.4 to determine serving equivalents for foods in the fat group.

TABLE 4.4

Fat—One Serving Size

1 tsp butter	1 tbsp cream cheese
1 tsp margarine	2 tbsp light cream cheese
1 tbsp diet margarine	2 tbsp sour cream
1 tsp mayonnaise	4 tbsp light sour cream
1 tbsp diet mayonnaise	2 tbsp coffee creamer (liquid)
1 tsp oil	
1 tbsp salad dressing	
2 tbsp diet salad dressing	

Young children are especially vulnerable to high-fat food consumption when you consider that many fast-food restaurants offer special incentives. Prepackaged meals typically include hamburgers, cheeseburgers, or batter-dipped chicken tenders with french fries and a choice of drink. The main attraction, however, is that these meals come with a special toy in the bag, usually depicting a character from the most recent children's animated films. Children not only want the toy, they want to collect *all* the toys featured in the collection, which lures them into a cycle of fast-food selections. What a difference it would make in our children's lifestyles if the prepackaged meal with a toy offered foods low in fat and high in nutrients rather than the opposite.

Summary

There are many benefits to establishing healthy eating patterns at an early age. First, proper nutrition provides a child with the necessary energy, nutrients, and building blocks to maintain an active lifestyle. Second, encouraging positive food choices may help a child continue similar behaviors into adulthood. Finally, although the effects of eating high-fat foods may not be evident for many years, food choices made in childhood have just as much impact on overall health as those made in adult life.

We must therefore counter high-fat, low-nutrient fast foods with alternatives that offer children optimum benefit for their health and fitness. We can do this by educating through example and by providing healthy meal and snack options that maximize muscle development and energy production, minimize fat accumulation, and truly appeal to a child. In so doing, youth will have the energy, enthusiasm, and equilibrium they need for a happy and healthy fitness future.

PART II

Equipment and Exercise

Free Weights

The equipment and exercises you will read about in this section represent only a few training options that are available for your youth strength-training program. We carefully chose several types of training equipment and the best strength-building exercises to provide you with a variety of safe and effective training options. Some exercises require special types of equipment, whereas others don't need anything at all. We believe that most modes of strength training can help children reach their training goals if they perform the exercises correctly. In this section we will highlight the advantages and disadvantages of free weights (dumbbells and barbells), weight machines, medicine balls, rubber tubing, and body-weight exercises. This chapter will begin with a discussion on safety, exercise technique, and free-weight training.

Before a child begins lifting weights, the strength-training area must be free of clutter and the room should be well lit and adequately ventilated. The equipment should be in an area that lets children move safely from one station to the next. If they use free weights, benches and weight racks should be nearby so that children do not have to walk too far with weights in their hands. This will reduce time spent carrying the weights and decrease traffic flow in the strength-training area. Parents and coaches need to designate a specific area in the weight room for multijoint free-weight lifts such as the squat and overhead press. Because the weight could slip out of a lifter's hands and result in injury, never allow children to perform a free-weight multijoint exercise near other children performing an exercise on the floor such as an abdominal curl. Also, children should always return barbells and dumbbells to the appropriate racks so they don't slip or trip on them. Following these sensible safety guidelines can reduce the likelihood of children getting hurt in the weight-training area.

When teaching a child a strength-training exercise, always focus on form and technique rather than the amount of weight he or she lifts. Thus you must completely understand how to perform an exercise before attempting to teach it to a child. Work with children in small groups, and always encourage children to ask questions and comment on the program. When teaching children a new exercise, ask them to stand in a semicircle around the exercise you are presenting to them. State the name of the exercise, and remind the children that the names of all exercises are posted in the exercise room. Then demonstrate five or six repetitions of the exercise, highlighting the muscles used, the importance of slow movements throughout a full range of motion, correct body positioning, and proper breathing. When teaching children a free-weight exercise, always start with a light weight, wooden stick, or plastic rod. This helps focus on form and technique while minimizing muscle soreness.

Next ask a child to demonstrate the proper exercise technique on a given exercise. Instruction can come from children as well as adults, and you may ask your regular participants to serve as junior instructors if they want to do so. Provide constructive feedback regarding the child's exercise performance, and upon completing the exercise gratefully acknowledge the child's willingness to demonstrate an exercise in front of his or her peers. Realize that learning most free-weight exercises requires coordination and concentration, and therefore limit the number of new exercises you add to a child's routine on any day. From our experience, attempting to add too many exercises to a child's routine at the same time slows the learning process and takes some fun out of the exercise program. Teach children something new every session, so they want to lift weights when they come to your class and therefore spend most of the time exercising and having fun.

When you teach children free-weight exercises, remember to demonstrate proper spotting techniques, which are essential for safe free-weight training. A spotter is a safety person who should be nearby to assist when a child is lifting a

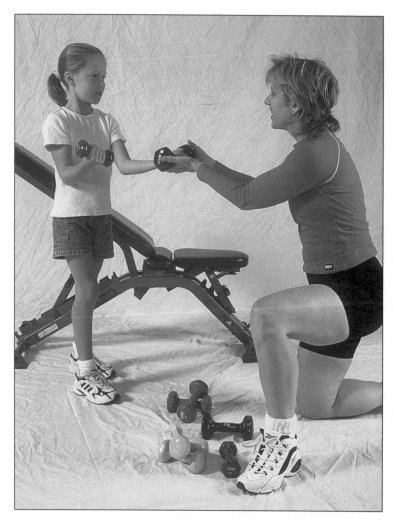

Always demonstrate correct body positioning.

weight over the body, when loss of balance may occur, or when learning a new exercise. Spotters should know proper exercise technique and should be able to handle the weight the child is lifting in case he or she needs assistance. Spotters should communicate with the lifter and should know how many repetitions the lifter will complete. Parents and coaches need to teach children about proper spotting techniques, as the purpose of correct spotting is to prevent injury. If children are too young to spot each other or if they have special needs and are unable to provide the necessary assistance, adults should serve as spotters. When working with a large class of children, it may be necessary to enlist the help of additional adults or separate the class into small groups.

Although different training modalities have proven safe and effective, we all need to appreciate that improper exercise technique on any type of equipment can place undue stress on a body part and may result in injury. This is important when performing free-weight exercises. For example, a child can injure the lower back if he or she does a rocking motion when performing a simple exercise such as the barbell curl. If this happens, it usually means that the child is lifting too much weight or isn't paying attention to the proper exercise technique. Without competent supervision and qualified instruction, children can develop poor exercise habits and injure themselves. You need to be sure that children understand the benefits as well as the risks inherent in this type of training. Constantly emphasize safety, and under no circumstances allow horseplay in the strength-training area. In our program, all youth fitness instructors demonstrate their commitment to safe strength training through their own actions in the strength-training area.

Training With Free Weights

Free-weight training refers to using barbells and dumbbells as well as various types of benches and racks. Barbells and dumbbells come in different shapes and sizes and may be adjustable or fixed. Most barbells sold in stores are about five feet long and weigh about 25 pounds. The adjustable barbells and dumbbells enable you to change the weight as needed by adding or removing weight plates, which you can secure to the bar by collars or locks. On the other hand, fixed barbells and dumbbells come in a predetermined weight that you cannot change. Because you don't have to change the weight for each exercise, fixed free weights can decrease the time of your workout. However, you will need to purchase several of them for all the different exercises in your workout. Depending on the age and ability of the children, these could include pairs of 2-, 3-, 5-, 8-, and 10-pound dumbbells. An economical approach is to purchase two adjustable dumbbells and several weight plates that are appropriate for your child's training level. Whatever type of equipment you use, keep in mind that it is important to increase the weight gradually as a child gets stronger. Generally, use one- to three-pound increases depending on the exercise.

Although most free-weight exercises we describe in this chapter only require dumbbells or barbells, you perform some free-weight exercises on a weight bench in a sitting or lying position. Weight benches are typically of two types: flat and incline. The adjustable incline weight bench is the most versatile because you can change it to various angles and seat positions. For general conditioning, any type of flat weight bench can work. As the training program progresses, you will need equipment such as a squat rack if you decide to perform the squat exercise with a barbell.

Free weights are inexpensive, and you can purchase them at most sporting good and fitness equipment stores. This type of equipment does not take up much room, and you can easily store it in a closet for safekeeping. Barbells and dumbbells allow unrestrained movement patterns, and therefore you can perform all free-weight exercises throughout their full range of motion. This not only helps enhance flexibility, but also improves muscle coordination because the child must learn to balance the weight in all directions (up, down, left, and right). Another advantage of using free weights compared with other types of equipment is that children of all sizes can use them and can perform hundreds of different exercises, including total-body movements. In addition, if one side of a child's body is weaker than the other, free weights allow you to restore muscle balance with appropriate training.

In general, you can consider free-weight training more technical than other modes of training, and therefore you must emphasize proper instruction and close supervision to be sure that the children perform the exercises correctly. Because the movements are not fixed (as on weight machines), children may be more likely to perform the exercise incorrectly. You also need to teach children how to hold dumbbells and weight plates correctly so they don't slip and fall out of their hands. During the first exercise session, it is important to show children how to hold free weights correctly with the thumb hooked under the bar and the knuckles on top of the bar. For some advanced free-weight exercises, such as the squat, children need to develop abdominal and lower-back strength before they add weight to the bar. This concern is important for sedentary children who typically have weak supporting muscles in their torsos. Our youth strength-training program begins with a basic program that includes abdominal and lower-back strengthening exercises in addition to exercises for the legs, chest, back, and arms. Over time we progress to advanced lifting techniques based on a child's exercise performance and willingness to try more challenging lifts.

Free-Weight Exercises

We have organized the free-weight exercises into two major sections: upper body and lower body. We have also listed the specific names of the primary muscle groups strengthened by each exercise. Understanding the muscles that you are training will help you design a balanced strength-training program. For example, overexercising the quadriceps (muscles on the front of the thigh) and underexercising the hamstrings (muscles on the back of the thigh) can make a child prone to injury. Children should begin strength training by focusing on all the major muscle groups to get the most from their workouts. Before children begin training with free weights, be sure to follow these safety guidelines:

- Knowledgeable adults should provide close supervision and instruction.
- If you use adjustable barbells and dumbbells, secure the weights with collars and load them evenly.
- Check the stability of benches and racks before you use them.

- Use a spotter when lifting a weight above your body, when loss of balance may occur, or when learning a new exercise.
- Always begin with a light weight and focus on learning the correct form of each exercise.
- If you cannot maintain proper exercise technique, stop the exercise and lower the weight.
- Remove weights from the floor to prevent slipping or tripping.
- When not being used, store free weights in a secure area so younger children don't get hurt.

Lower-Body Exercises

DUMBBELL SQUAT

MUSCLES

- Quadriceps, hamstrings, gluteals

PROCEDURE

- Begin by grasping a dumbbell in each hand, and stand erect with feet about hip-width apart and toes pointing slightly outward. Hold the dumbbells so they hang straight down at the sides of your body.
- Slowly bend your ankles, knees, and hips until your thighs are parallel to the floor. Keep your back flat, head up, and eyes fixed straight ahead.
- Return to starting position by slowly straightening your knees and hips.

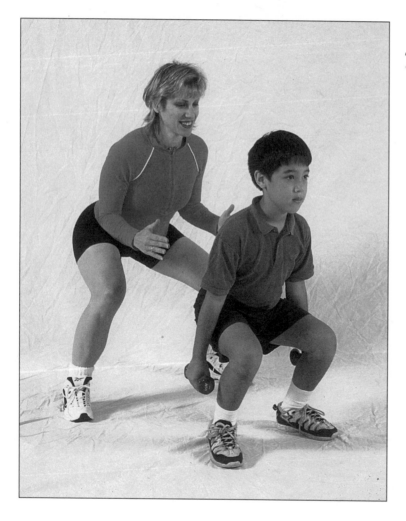

Technique Tips

- Your knees should follow a slightly outward pattern of the feet. Do not let the knees cave in.
- Inhale during the downward phase of the exercise and exhale during the upward phase.
- Avoid bouncing out of the bottom position.
- Concentrate on keeping your head up and chest out. Avoid excessive forward lean.
- Beginners may find it easier to learn this exercise by positioning their upper back and buttocks against a wall for support (i.e., slide up and down a wall).
- You can also perform this exercise with a barbell, providing skilled instruction and supervision are available.
- It is important that an adult spotter be nearby to provide assistance if needed.

BARBELL SQUAT

MUSCLES

- Quadriceps, hamstrings, gluteals

PROCEDURE

- Grasp the barbell with an overhand grip while it is on the rack.
- Your hands should be wider than shoulder-width apart, and the barbell should rest on your shoulders and upper trapezius muscle, not on your neck.
- Lift the bar off the rack. Keep your back straight, eyes looking forward, and feet slightly wider than shoulder-width apart.
- Slowly bend your knees and hips until your thighs are parallel to the floor. Keep your heels in contact with the floor.
- Return to the starting position by straightening your knees and hips.
- When you have completed the desired number of repetitions, walk the barbell back to the rack.

Technique Tips

- Inhale during the lowering phase and exhale during the lifting phase.
- Your back should remain upright during this exercise. Excessive forward lean places undue stress on your lower back and may result in an injury.
- A spotter should stand directly behind the lifter during this exercise.

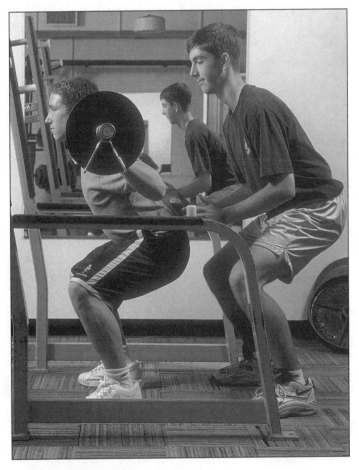

DUMBBELL LUNGE

MUSCLES

- Quadriceps, hamstrings, gluteals

PROCEDURE

- Begin by grasping a dumbbell in each hand. Stand erect with feet about hip-width apart, and hold the dumbbells so they hang straight down at the sides of your body. Look straight forward.
- Take a long step forward with your right leg; bend the knee of the right leg and lower your body. The thigh of the right leg should be parallel to the floor, and the right knee should be over the ankle of the right foot. Bend the left knee slightly.

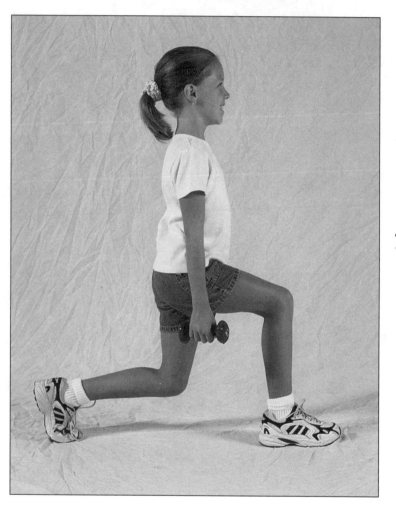

- Return to the starting position by pushing off the floor with the right leg. Take one or two steps backward to the starting position. Repeat with the opposite leg.
- Keep your head up, back upright, and shoulders over the hips.

Technique Tips

- This exercise requires balance and coordination. Begin with just your body weight to learn proper form.
- Keep your head up, back upright, and shoulders over the hips.
- Inhale during the forward phase of the exercise and exhale during the return phase.
- Avoid using upper-torso momentum to return to the starting position. Concentrate on keeping your back upright throughout the exercise.

DUMBBELL SIDE LUNGE

MUSCLES

- Quadriceps, hamstrings, gluteals, hip abductors and adductors

PROCEDURE

- Begin by grasping a dumbbell in each hand. Stand erect with your feet about shoulder-width apart, and hold the dumbbells in front of your body. Look straight forward.
- Lunge to the side of your body with one leg while holding the dumbbells in front of your body.
- Point your toes slightly to the side as you step out.
- Bend your knee until your thigh is parallel to the floor.
- Then push yourself to the starting position.
- Repeat with the opposite leg.

Technique Tips

- Inhale as you lunge to the side and exhale as you return to the starting position.
- Keep your head up and facing forward during this exercise.
- This exercise requires balance and coordination. Begin with just your body weight to learn the proper form.

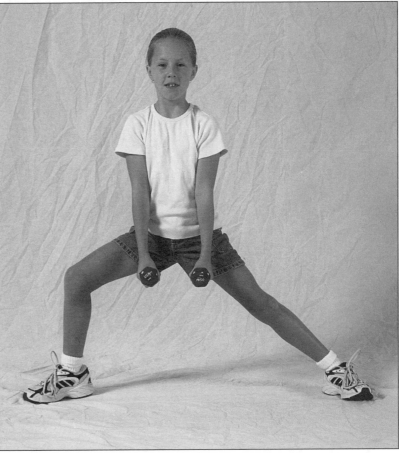

DUMBBELL STEP-UP

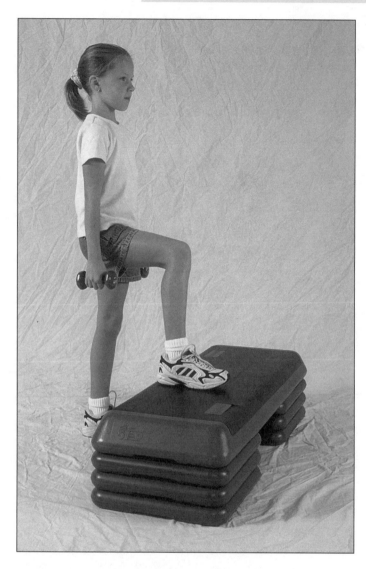

MUSCLES

- Quadriceps, gluteals, hip extensors

PROCEDURE

- Begin by grasping a dumbbell in each hand, and stand erect with feet about hip-width apart. Hold the dumbbells so they hang straight down at the sides of your body. Look straight forward.
- Begin with your right leg, and step onto a bench that is about knee height. Lift your body with your right leg. Bring the knee of your left leg up.
- Slowly lower your body by stepping back down to the starting position. Repeat with the opposite leg.

Technique Tips

- This exercise requires balance and coordination. Begin with just your body weight to learn proper form.
- Exhale during the upward phase of the exercise and inhale during the downward phase.
- Concentrate on keeping the torso upright during this exercise.
- Before starting, check to be sure the bench is stable and secure.

DUMBBELL HEEL RAISE

MUSCLES

- Gastrocnemius, soleus

PROCEDURE

- Begin by grasping a dumbbell in the right hand. Place the full ball of the right foot on a board or step with the heel off the surface. Wrap the left foot behind the right ankle. Use the free left hand for balance by holding onto the wall or bench.

- Raise up onto the right toe as high as possible; then slowly lower the heel as far as comfortable. Complete the assigned number of repetitions, and repeat with the opposite leg.

Technique Tips

- Inhale during the lowering phase of the exercise and exhale during the upward phase.

- Concentrate on keeping your torso and knees straight to avoid upper-leg involvement.

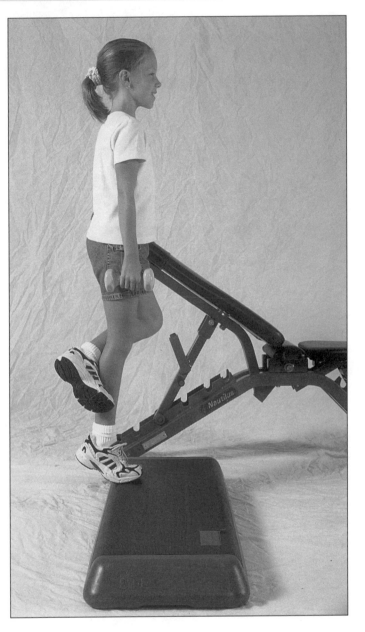

BARBELL HEEL RAISE

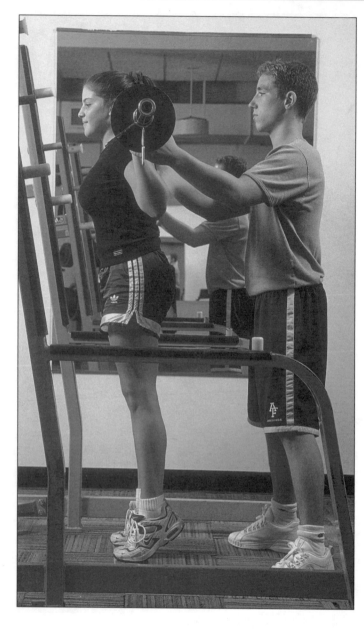

MUSCLES

- Gastrocnemius, soleus

PROCEDURE

- Grasp barbell with a wider than shoulder-width grip, and position barbell across your shoulders and upper trapezius, not on your neck.
- Stand erect with your feet about shoulder-width apart. Keep your torso and knees straight.
- Slowly raise up on the toes as high as possible; then return to starting position.

Technique Tips

- Exhale as you lift the weight and inhale on the return movement.
- To increase the range of motion, stand with the balls of your feet on a board about one to two inches high.
- A spotter should stand behind the lifter in case the lifter needs assistance.

TOE RAISE

MUSCLES

- Tibialis anterior

PROCEDURE

- Sit on the edge of a high bench with your legs hanging straight down. Attach one end of a looped rope near the toe and ball area of one foot. Attach a light weight to the other end of the rope, and let the weight hang freely.
- Lower the toe and ball area of your foot as far as possible.
- Lift the weight by raising the toe and ball area of your foot as high as possible.
- Pause briefly, then slowly lower the weight to the starting position.

Technique Tips

- Exhale as you lift the weight and inhale as you lower it.
- You need only a light weight for this exercise because these are small muscles.
- Note that you cannot raise your foot much farther than the horizontal position. Thus it is important to lower the toe and ball area of your foot as much as possible to perform this exercise through the maximum range of motion.

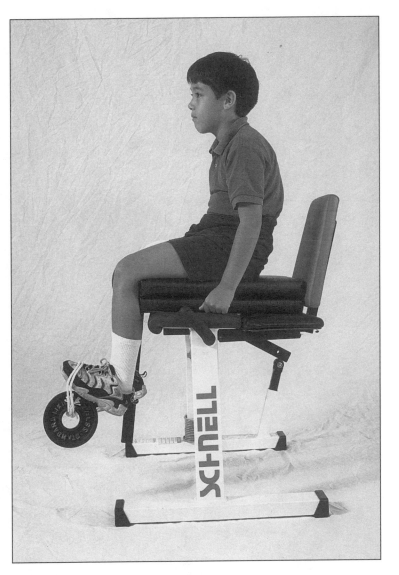

Upper-Body Exercises

DUMBBELL CHEST PRESS

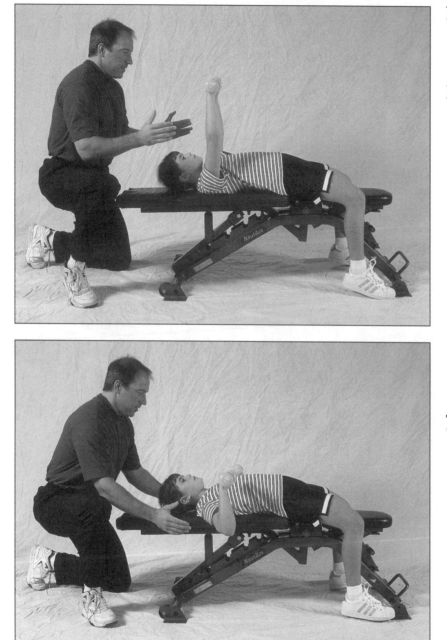

MUSCLES

- Pectoralis major, anterior deltoid, triceps

PROCEDURE

- Grasp a dumbbell in each hand. Lie on your back on a bench with your feet flat on the floor. If your feet don't reach the floor, use a stable board to accommodate size. Hold the dumbbells at arm's length over the chest area with palms facing away from your body.
- Slowly bend your elbows and lower the dumbbells to the outside of the chest area.
- Press the dumbbells upward until you fully extend both arms.

Technique Tips

- Inhale during the lowering phase of the exercise and exhale during the upward phase.
- Keep your head, shoulders, and buttocks in contact with the bench during this exercise. Do not twist or arch your body.
- Keep the dumbbells above your chest and not above your face.
- It is important that a spotter is nearby to provide assistance if needed. A spotter can place his or her hands on the child's wrists to teach proper dumbbell exercise technique or complete a repetition.
- You can also perform this exercise with a barbell, providing skilled instruction and supervision are available. If you perform this exercise with a barbell, an adult spotter must be nearby to provide assistance if necessary.

DUMBBELL INCLINE PRESS

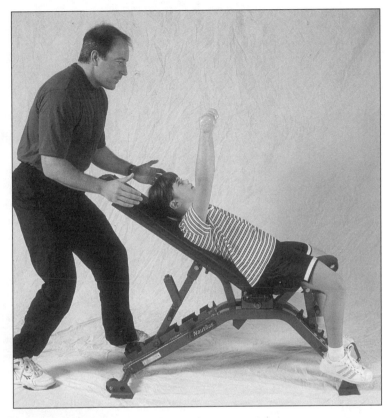

This exercise is the same as the dumbbell chest press except you perform it on an inclined bench, typically angled between 30 to 45 degrees.

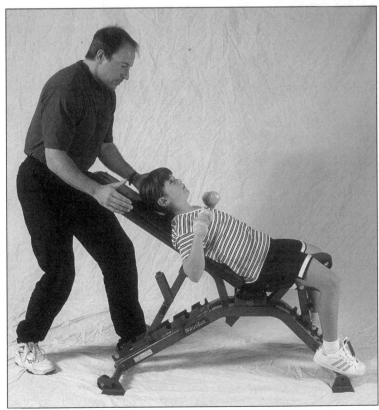

Start with the dumbbells above the chin. Finish with the dumbbells just above the upper chest.

BARBELL BENCH PRESS

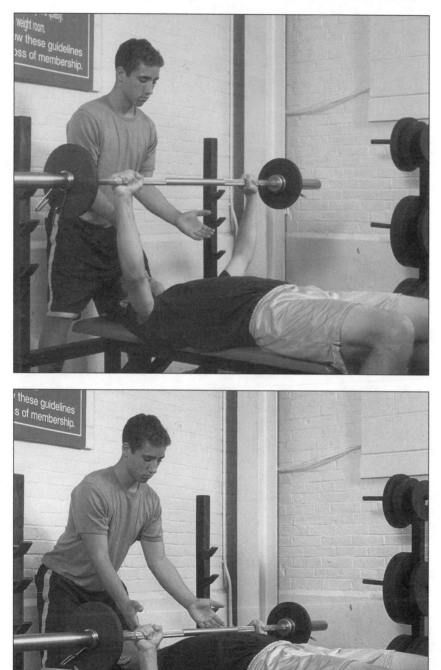

MUSCLES

- Pectoralis major, anterior deltoid, triceps

PROCEDURE

- Lie on your back with your feet flat on the floor. Grasp the barbell with a wider than shoulder-width grip. Hold the barbell at arm's length above your upper-chest area.
- Slowly lower the barbell to the middle of your chest. Pause briefly, then press the barbell to the starting position. During the movement, the upper arms should be about 45 to 60 degrees from the torso.

Technique Tips

- Inhale as you lower the weight and exhale as you lift it.
- A spotter should be behind the lifter's head and should assist the lifter with getting the barbell into the starting position and returning the barbell to the rack when finished. Impress on young weight trainers the importance of a spotter during the exercise because the bar is pressed over the lifter's face, neck, and chest.
- Learn this exercise with an unloaded barbell or long stick.
- Do not bounce the barbell off the chest, and do not lift your buttocks off the bench during this exercise.
- Avoid hitting the upright supports by positioning your body about three inches from the supports before you start.

DUMBBELL CHEST FLY

MUSCLES

- Pectoralis major, anterior deltoid

PROCEDURE

- Grasp a dumbbell in each hand. Lie on your back on a bench with your feet flat on the floor. If your feet don't reach the floor, use a stable lift to accommodate size. Hold the dumbbells at arm's length over the chest area with your palms facing each other and arms slightly bent.

- Slowly lower the dumbbells until your upper arms are parallel to the floor. You should feel a gentle stretch across your chest.

- Lift the dumbbells to starting position, keeping your elbows slightly bent.

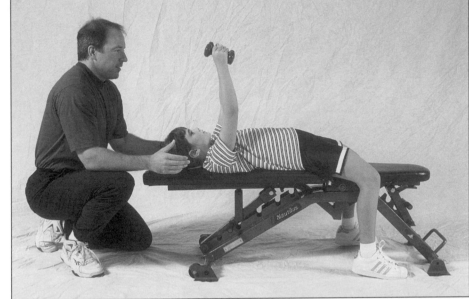

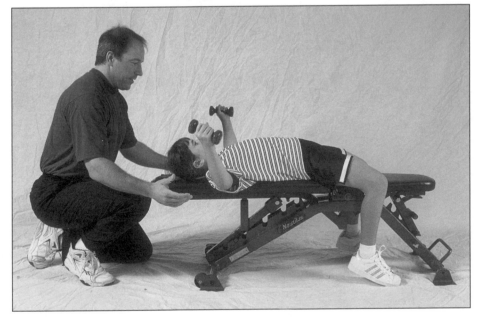

Technique Tips

- Inhale during the lowering phase of the exercise and exhale during the upward phase.

- Keep head, shoulders, and buttocks in contact with the bench during this exercise. Do not twist or arch your body.

- Keep the dumbbells above your chest and not above your face.

- It is important that a spotter is nearby to provide assistance if needed. A spotter can place his or her hands on the child's wrists to teach proper exercise technique or complete a repetition.

DUMBBELL ONE-ARM ROW

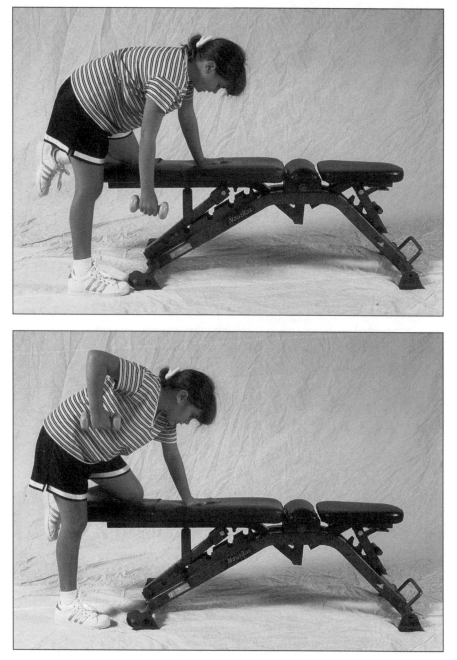

MUSCLES

- Latissimus dorsi, biceps

PROCEDURE

- Grasp a dumbbell in the right hand with the palm facing the side of the body, and place the left hand and left knee on the bench. Bend over at the waist so the upper body and lower back are parallel (flat) to the floor. Support the body on the bench, and keep the back flat from the shoulders to the hips. Lower the dumbbell toward the floor so you fully extend the right arm.

- Slowly pull the dumbbell upward until it reaches the side of the chest area. Then lower the dumbbell back to the straight-arm position. Perform the assigned number of repetitions; then switch the supporting posture and exercise your left side.

Technique Tips

- Exhale during the pulling phase of the exercise and inhale during the lowering phase.

- The legs and nonexercising arm should remain stationary during the exercise. The lower back should not rotate during this exercise.

- For variation, you can perform this exercise with the elbow pointing away from the body (palm toward feet) during the lifting motion.

DUMBBELL PULLOVER

MUSCLES

- Latissimus dorsi

PROCEDURE

- Grasp one dumbbell with both hands, and lie on a flat bench with your arms extended over your chest area. Secure your grip by cupping both hands around one end of the dumbbell.

- Slowly lower the dumbbell behind your head toward the floor as far as comfortable. Maintain a slight bend in your elbows. Then slowly return to starting position.

Technique Tips

- Inhale as you lower the weight and exhale as you lift it.

- A spotter should kneel directly behind the lifter's head during this exercise and provide assistance if necessary.

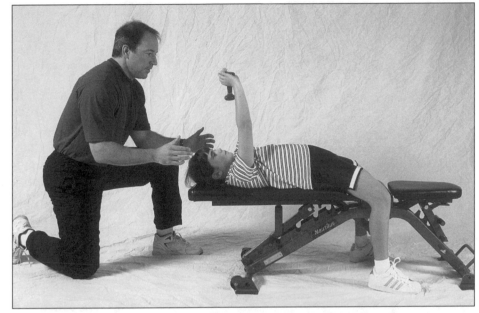

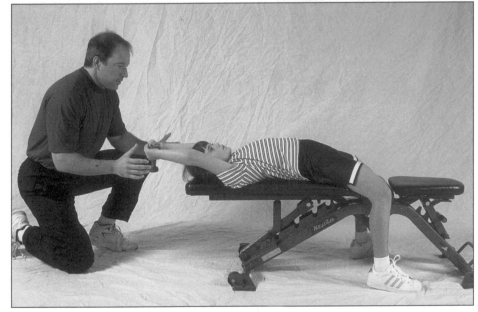

- Because the dumbbell is over the head of the lifter, begin with a light weight and gradually increase the load. We recommend a solid dumbbell (rather than a dumbbell with plates and collars) for this exercise.

DUMBBELL UPRIGHT ROW

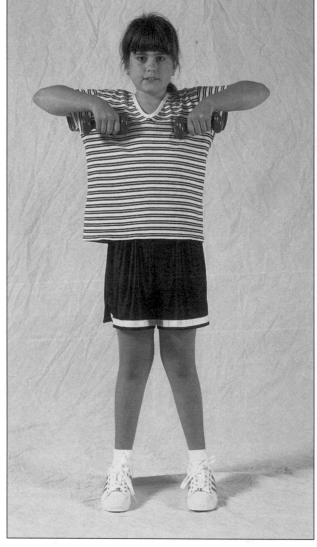

MUSCLES

- Deltoids, upper trapezius, biceps

PROCEDURE

- Begin by grasping a dumbbell in each hand, and stand erect with feet about hip-width apart. Hold the dumbbells so they hang straight down in front of your body with your palms facing your body. The dumbbells should be closer than shoulder-width apart.
- Slowly pull both dumbbells upward to the height of the upper chest; then lower them to the starting position.

Technique Tips

- Exhale during the lifting phase of the exercise and inhale during the lowering phase.
- Stand erect and keep the dumbbells close to your body during this exercise.
- At the top of the movement the elbows should be higher than the shoulders.
- You can also perform this exercise with a barbell, providing skilled instruction and supervision are available.

DUMBBELL OVERHEAD PRESS

MUSCLES

- Deltoids, upper trapezius, triceps

PROCEDURE

- Begin by grasping a dumbbell in each hand, and stand erect with feet about hip-width apart. Hold the dumbbells at shoulder height with your palms facing away from your body.
- Slowly push both dumbbells upward until you fully extend both arms over the shoulders; then lower the dumbbells to the starting position.

Technique Tips

- This exercise requires balance and coordination. Begin with a light weight to learn proper form.
- Exhale during the lifting phase of the exercise and inhale during the lowering phase.
- Stand erect and keep your lower back straight by contracting your abdominal and lower-back muscles.
- You can also perform this exercise while sitting on an adjustable incline bench or chair, which can provide back support and stability.
- You can also perform this exercise with a barbell, providing skilled instruction and supervision are available.
- It is important that a spotter is nearby to provide assistance if needed. A spotter can place his or her hands on the child's wrists to teach proper exercise technique or complete a repetition.

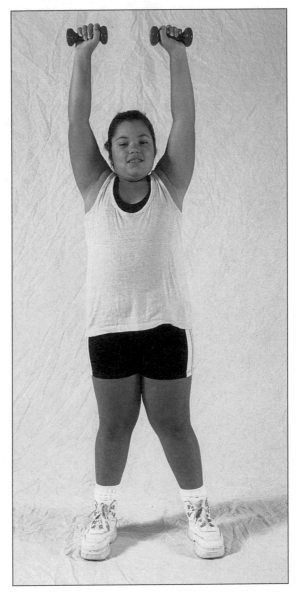

DUMBBELL LATERAL RAISE

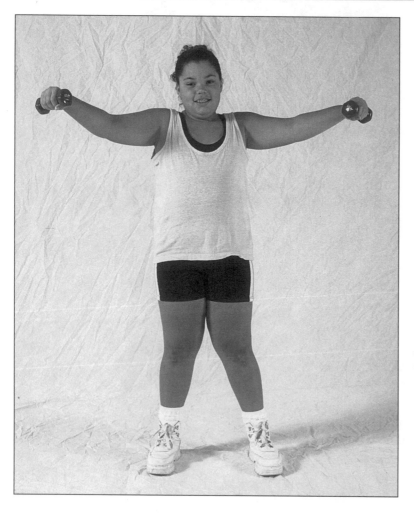

MUSCLES

- Deltoids

PROCEDURE

- Begin by grasping a dumbbell in each hand, and stand erect with your arms extended at your sides and palms facing your outer thighs. Your elbows should be slightly bent, and your feet should be about hip-width apart.
- Slowly lift both dumbbells upward and sideward until your arms are level with your shoulders (arms parallel to floor). Keep your elbows slightly bent, and return to starting position.

Technique Tips

- Exhale during the lifting phase of the exercise and inhale during the lowering phase.
- Stand erect and keep your lower back straight by contracting your abdominal and lower-back muscles.
- Don't raise your arms higher than parallel to the floor.

DUMBBELL SHRUG

MUSCLES

- Upper trapezius

PROCEDURE

- Begin by grasping a dumbbell in each hand, and stand erect with your arms extended at your sides and palms facing your outer thighs. Your arms should be fully extended, and your feet should be about hip-width apart.
- Slowly elevate (shrug) both shoulders toward the ears as high as possible; then lower both dumbbells to the starting position.

Technique Tips

- Exhale during the lifting phase of the exercise and inhale during the lowering phase.
- Stand erect and keep your lower back straight by contracting your abdominal and lower-back muscles.
- Don't bend your elbows while lifting the weights.

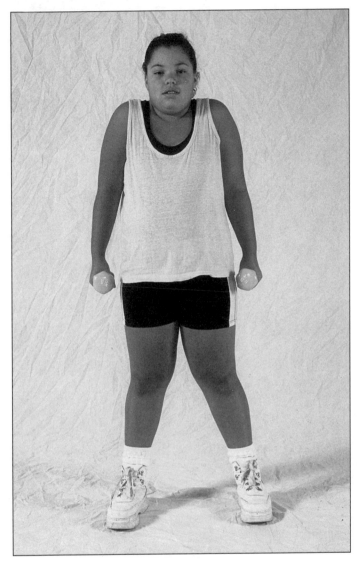

DUMBBELL
SHOULDER EXTERNAL ROTATION

MUSCLES

- Rotator cuff musculature

PROCEDURE

- Lie on your side in a comfortable position. Hold a light dumbbell with the top hand, and maintain the elbow in a 90-degree angle. Hold the upper arm against the side of your body. Use your other arm to support your head.
- Rotate your forearm out and up without letting your elbow move away from your body. Then slowly return to the starting position.

Technique Tips

- Exhale as you lift the weight and inhale as you lower it.
- This is a lightweight exercise. Start with a two- or three-pound dumbbell, and increase in one-pound increments.
- Keep your arm pressed against your body during this exercise.
- You can also perform this exercise in the standing position by using rubber tubing attached to a sturdy object or a cable attached to appropriate resistance.

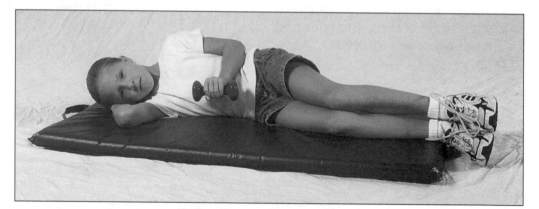

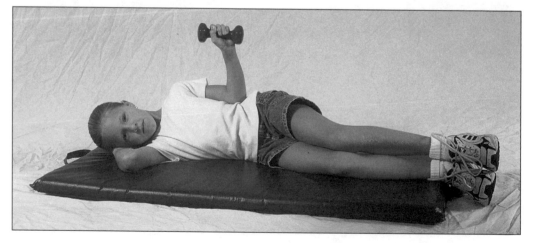

DUMBBELL
SHOULDER INTERNAL ROTATION

MUSCLES

- Rotator cuff musculature

PROCEDURE

- Lie on your back in a comfortable position. Hold a light dumbbell with one hand, and maintain the elbow in a 90-degree angle. Hold your upper arm on the floor against the side of your body and your forearm perpendicular to the floor.
- Slowly lower the dumbbell toward the floor by rotating your shoulder. Then return to the starting position.

Technique Tips

- Inhale as you lower the weight and exhale as you lift it.
- This is a lightweight exercise. Start with a two- or three-pound dumbbell, and increase in one-pound increments.
- Keep the elbow pressed against your body during this exercise.
- You can also perform this exercise in the standing position by using rubber tubing attached to a sturdy object or a cable attached to appropriate resistance.

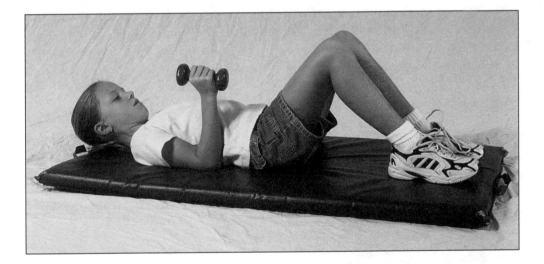

DUMBBELL BICEPS CURL

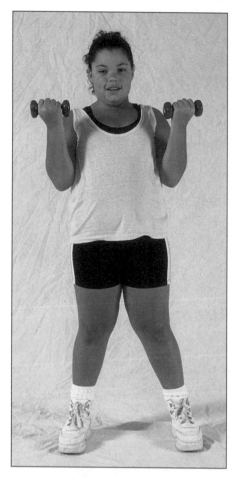

MUSCLES

• Biceps

PROCEDURE

• Begin by grasping a dumbbell in each hand, and stand erect with your arms extended at your sides and palms facing forward. Fully extend your arms, and place your feet about hip-width apart.

• Slowly curl both dumbbells upward toward your shoulders until your palms face the chest. Then lower both dumbbells to the starting position.

Technique Tips

• Exhale during the lifting phase of the exercise and inhale during the lowering phase.

• Stand erect and keep your lower back straight by contracting your abdominal and lower-back muscles.

• If necessary stand with your back against the wall to prevent upper-body torso movement.

• You can also perform this exercise while sitting on an adjustable incline bench, which can provide back support and stability.

• You can also perform this exercise with a barbell, providing skilled instruction and supervision are available.

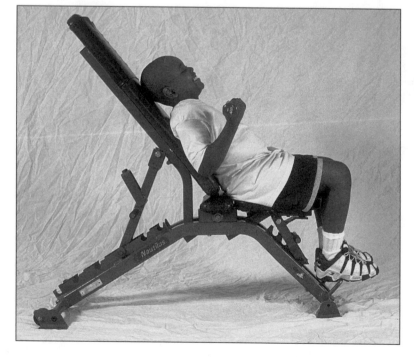

DUMBBELL INCLINE BICEPS CURL

This exercise is the same as the dumbbell biceps curl, except you perform it on an inclined bench, typically angled between 45 to 60 degrees.

DUMBBELL TRICEPS KICKBACK

MUSCLES

- Triceps

PROCEDURE

- Grasp a dumbbell in the right hand with the palm facing the side of the body, and place the left hand and left knee on the bench. Bend over at the waist so the upper body and lower back are parallel (flat) to the floor. Bend the right elbow to 90 degrees so the right forearm is perpendicular to the floor. Support the body on the bench, and keep the back flat from the shoulders to the hips.

- Slowly straighten the right arm until it is fully extended; then return to starting position. Perform the assigned number of repetitions; then switch your supporting posture and exercise your left arm.

Technique Tips

- Exhale during the lifting phase of the exercise and inhale during the lowering phase.

- Only the elbow and forearm should move during this exercise. The legs and non-exercising arm should remain stationary and the lower back should not rotate.

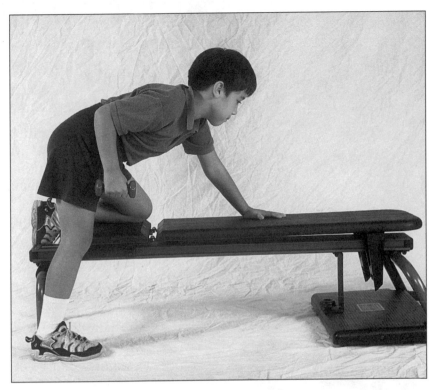

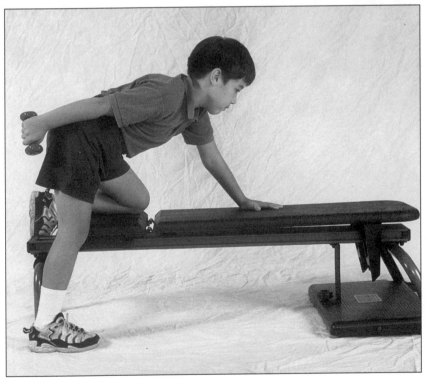

DUMBBELL TRICEPS OVERHEAD EXTENSION

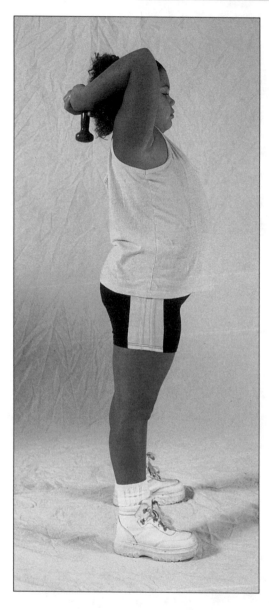

MUSCLES

- Triceps

PROCEDURE

- Grasp one dumbbell with both hands and extend your arms overhead. Interlace your fingers under the dumbbell. Keep your torso erect and eyes facing forward. Your upper arms remain perpendicular to the floor during this exercise.
- Slowly bend your elbows and lower the dumbbell behind your head. Pause briefly, then return to starting position.

Technique Tips

- Inhale during the lowering phase and exhale during the lifting phase.
- Maintain an erect posture during this exercise. Avoid leaning forward or backward. Keep your elbows pointing upward as you lower and raise the dumbbell.

DUMBBELL WRIST CURL

MUSCLES

- Wrist flexors

PROCEDURE

- Begin by kneeling on the floor with the forearms resting on a bench. Grasp a dumbbell in each hand in a palms-up position so the wrists just hang over the bench.
- Slowly flex the fingers and the wrists as high as possible while keeping the forearms flat on the bench; then return to starting position.

Technique Tips

- The entire forearm should remain in contact with the bench during this exercise. Only the fingers and wrists should move.
- You can also perform this exercise with one dumbbell at a time or with a barbell, providing skilled instruction and supervision are available.

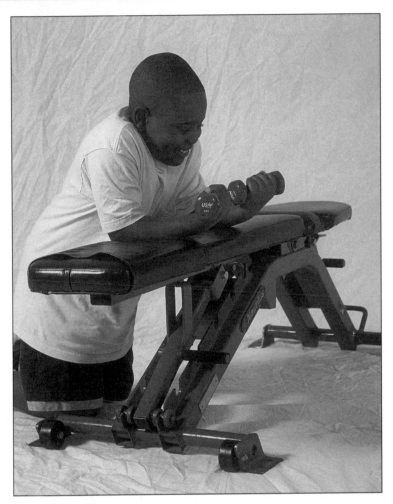

DUMBBELL WRIST EXTENSION

MUSCLES

- Wrist extensors

PROCEDURE

- Begin by kneeling on the floor with the forearms resting on a bench. Grasp a dumbbell in each hand in a palms-down position, and place the palm side of the forearms on the bench so the wrists just hang over the bench.
- Slowly lift the fingers and the wrists as high as possible while keeping the forearms flat on the bench; then return to starting position.

Technique Tips

- The entire forearm should remain in contact with the bench during this exercise. Only the fingers and wrists should move.
- Because this muscle group is weak, begin with a light weight.
- You can also perform this exercise with one dumbbell at a time or with a barbell, providing skilled instruction and supervision are available.

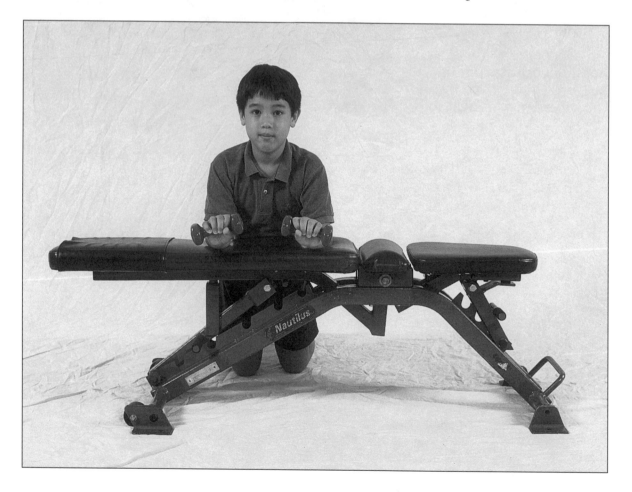

WRIST ROLLER

MUSCLES

- Wrist flexors and extensors

PROCEDURE

- Grasp the handle of the wrist roller with your palms facing downward. Stand erect with your elbows bent slightly.
- Roll up the string on the bar until the weight reaches the uppermost part. Then slowly unroll the string.

Technique Tips

- Start with a light weight, and gradually increase the resistance as strength improves.
- Vary the exercise by starting with the string between you and the roller and with the string on the opposite side of the roller.
- As you rotate the roller clockwise, you strengthen the wrist flexors. As you rotate the roller counterclockwise, you strengthen the wrist extensors.

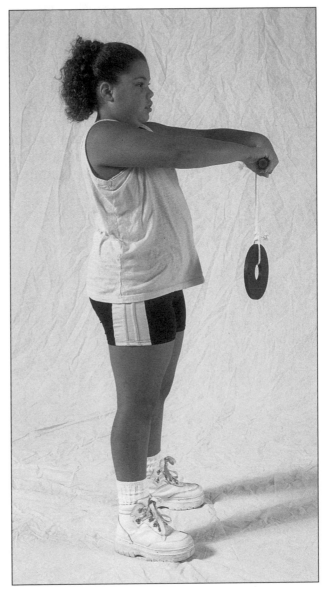

Summary

Strength training with barbells and dumbbells can be safe and effective provided that children are given an opportunity to learn proper exercise technique. Take the time to demonstrate each exercise to all participants and then provide constructive feedback regarding each child's exercise performance. We encourage children to ask questions and realize that learning free weight exercises requires coordination and concentration. Unlike some other modes of training, barbells and dumbbells allow unrestrained movement patterns, and therefore children of all sizes can use them and hundreds of different exercises can be performed. Further, free weights are relatively inexpensive and are readily available at most sporting good and fitness equipment stores.

6

Weight Machines

The growing interest in strength training by adults and children has led to the development of different types of weight machines, from single-station units to multipurpose machines with 5 to 10 exercise stations. In general, weight machines are easy to use because they provide a fixed movement pattern for each exercise and most provide support for your body. Because some weight machines allow you to train specific muscle groups, you can also use them to isolate a muscle that may be prone to injury. Further, well-designed weight machines attempt to match the weight to your strength by means of a cam or other accommodating resistance device. That is, some machines allow the lifter to maintain a constant level of exertion throughout each repetition. Although weight machines are more expensive than other types of strength-training equipment, they enable you to perform some strength-building exercises, such as the leg curl and front pulldown that you can't do with free weights.

For many years weight machines were made only for adults. Although our big teenagers could properly fit into these machines, some young weight trainers were too short. Thus small children could not position themselves properly on the machines, and they could not perform most exercises throughout the full range of motion. Because children's limbs are shorter than those of adults, improper positioning could result in an injury if a child's arm or leg slipped off the

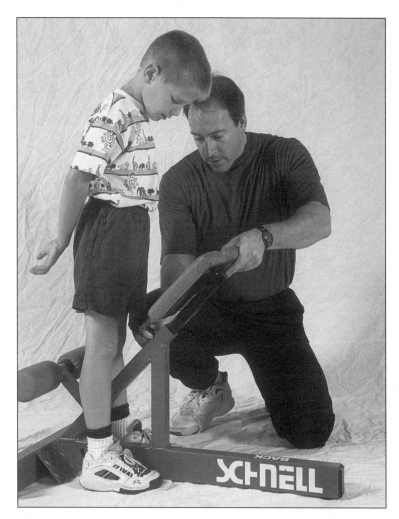

Due to differences in body size, adjust equipment to ensure proper fit.

pad or if the pad moved during the performance of an exercise. Even though you can easily modify some machines, such as the shoulder press, with a few seat pads, we need to account for proper positioning of all body parts and machine-to-body relationships. Just because you can adjust the seat does not mean that a child can properly fit into the machine with desirable biomechanical alignments.

In all cases, you must do modifications to adult-sized equipment carefully so you never compromise the safety of the young lifter. When deciding on equipment needs, realize that children must fit into a weight machine properly for the biomechanical requirements of the muscle action to match the training equipment. Above all, if you cannot properly adapt a weight machine to fit the child, do not use that machine. Remember that safety is the most important issue. Generally, you can modify adult machines by adding seat pads beneath the hips or behind the back so the children can perform the exercise in the desired movement range.

Fortunately, several companies have started to manufacture youth strength-training equipment that is durable, versatile, easy to use, and safe. This type of equipment is similar in design to adult-sized machines, but it is scaled down to fit smaller bodies. Single-station units and multistation machines that use pin-operated weight stacks or weight plates are available. One great advantage of child-sized weight machines is that the weight stacks are designed to increase in only five-pound increments. If this is too heavy, you can add specially designed one- and two-and-one-half-pound plates to the weight stack as needed. A potential problem with some types of adult weight machines is that the initial weight is too much for a child, or the 10- to 20-pound increases in weight are too large. Although there are many different types of adult- and child-sized weight machines, the structure and function of a particular exercise, such as the leg press, is the same on all machines. Thus you can easily adapt the exercises we describe in this chapter to your weight machines.

Training on Weight Machines

Despite the claims of some weight-machine manufacturers, we believe that most types of strength-training equipment can be safe and effective for children, provided that they follow appropriate guidelines. In our view, caring and competent instruction and supervision are more important than the type of equipment you have in your home or at your gym. If you have access to adult-sized weight machines, make the necessary modifications to ensure proper fit. Remember that, in many cases, simply adjusting the seat height does not necessarily mean that a child can safely fit onto a piece of equip-

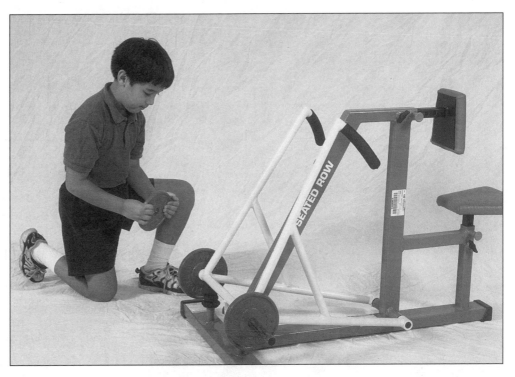

Always carry weight plates with two hands.

ment. No matter what type of weight machines you use—adult or child size—take the following safety steps before and during your exercise sessions:

- Check for frayed cables, worn chains, and loose pads.
- If the machines are plate loaded, always carry the plates with two hands.
- Adjust seats and pads as needed.
- If you use a selector pin, be sure that you insert it all the way into the weight stack.
- Keep hands away from chains, belts, pulleys, and cams.
- Never place your hands or feet between the weight stacks.
- Concentrate on lifting and lowering the weights slowly and under control. Do not drop the weight to the starting position.

Weight-Machine Exercises

We organized the weight-machine exercises in this chapter into two major sections: upper body and lower body. We also note the names of the primary muscles strengthened by each exercise. This format should make it easy for parents and coaches to choose exercises that train all the major muscle groups. Remember that it is important to create balance in your strength-training workout so you exercise opposing muscle groups equally. For example, if you perform a chest exercise, you should also perform an exercise for your upper back. Take the time to learn the different muscle groups, as this will help you get the most from your workouts.

Lower-Body Exercises

LEG PRESS

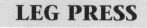

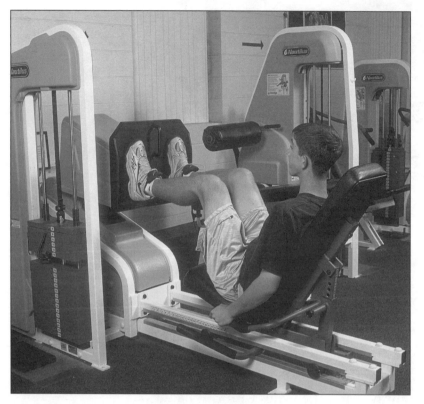

MUSCLES

- Quadriceps, hamstrings, gluteals

PROCEDURE

- Adjust the back pad so you flex your knees to 90 degrees.
- Sit with your back firmly against the back pad. Place your feet on the footpad, in line with your knees and hips. Grip the handles to keep your buttocks on the seat throughout the exercise.
- Slowly press evenly with both feet until you almost extend, but don't lock, your knees.
- Return to starting position by slowly bending your knees. Then begin the forward movement before the weight touches the stack.

Technique Tips

- Exhale during the pressing movement and inhale during the return movement.
- Do not lock your knees in the extended position.

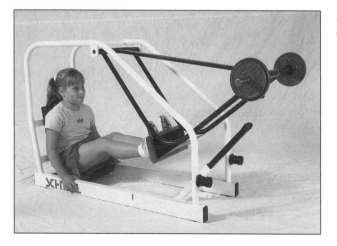

For Younger Athletes

- Place feet firmly on the foot pad.
- Keep your back pressed against the seat.
- Keep hands away from moving parts.

LEG EXTENSION

MUSCLES

- Quadriceps

PROCEDURE

- Adjust the back pad so your knees are in line with the machine's axis of rotation. Position your ankles behind the roller pad.
- Sit erect with your knees bent about 90 degrees and your back firmly against the pad. Grip both handles.
- Lift the roller pad upward until you fully extend your knees.
- Return to the starting position by slowly bending your knees. Then begin the upward movement before the weight touches the stack.

Technique Tips

- Exhale during the lifting movement and inhale during the lowering movement.
- Grip the handles firmly to keep your buttocks on the seat throughout the exercise.

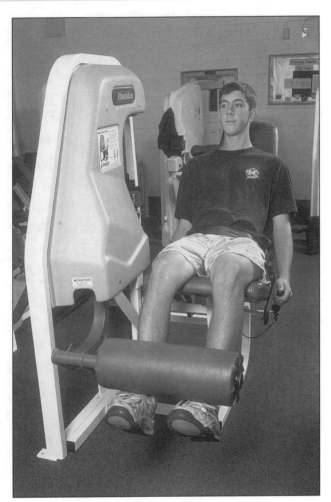

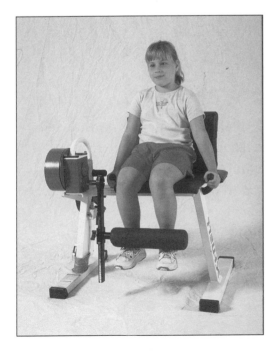

For Younger Athletes

- Upper body should not move during exercise.
- Adjust ankle pad to child's length.
- Grasp handles throughout exercise.

LEG CURL

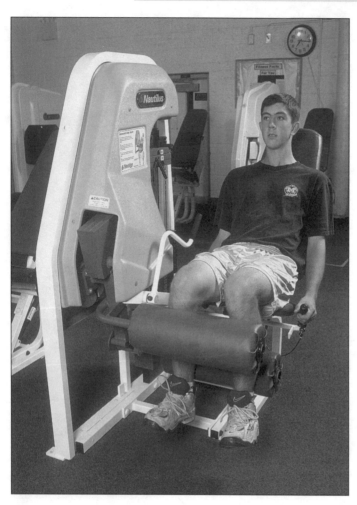

MUSCLES

- Hamstrings

PROCEDURE

- Adjust the back pad so your knees are in line with the machine's axis of rotation. Position your lower legs between the roller pads.
- Sit erect with your knees straight and your back firmly against the pad. Grip both handles.
- Pull the roller pads downward until your knees are bent about 90 degrees.
- Return to the starting position by slowly straightening your knees. Begin the downward movement before the weight touches the stack.

Technique Tips

- Exhale during the lifting movement and inhale during the lowering movement.
- Keep your hips and back in contact with the seat during this exercise.
- Learn this exercise with a light weight at first.

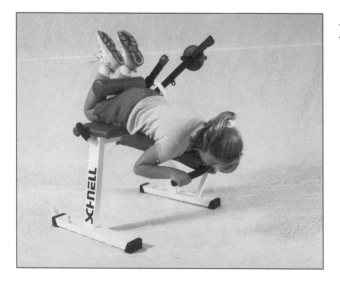

For Younger Athletes

- Upper body should not move during exercise.
- Adjust ankle pad to child's length.
- Grasp handles throughout the exercise.
- Keep head in line with the body at all times.

HIP ADDUCTION

MUSCLES

- Hip adductors

PROCEDURE

- Sit on the machine with your shoulders and back against the pad. Place your legs on the rungs of the machine with your ankles on the supports.
- Adjust the movement lever to its appropriate starting position. Grasp the handles.
- Slowly squeeze your legs together as far as possible; then return to starting position.

Technique Tips

- Exhale as you squeeze your legs together and inhale as you bring your legs apart.
- Do not begin this exercise from an overstretched position.
- You can also perform this exercise on a standing hip adduction machine. Face the machine and adjust the pad to just above knee level.

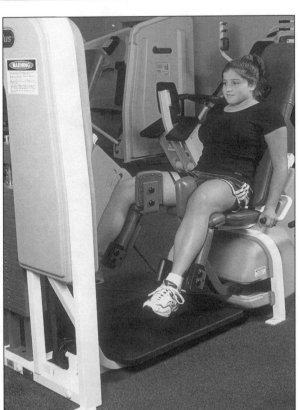

HIP ABDUCTION

MUSCLES

- Hip abductors

PROCEDURE

- Sit on the machine with your shoulders and back against the pad. Place your legs on the rungs of the machine with your ankles on the supports.
- Slowly pull your legs apart as far as possible; then return to starting position.

Technique Tips

- Exhale as you pull your legs apart and inhale as you bring your legs together.
- You can also perform this exercise on a standing hip abduction machine. Face the machine and adjust the pad to just above knee level.

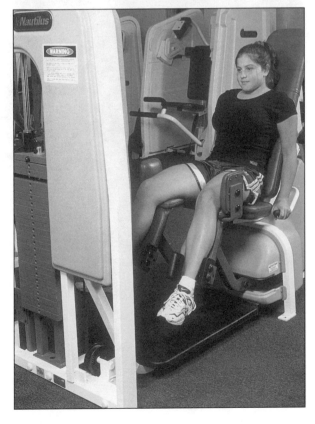

HEEL RAISE

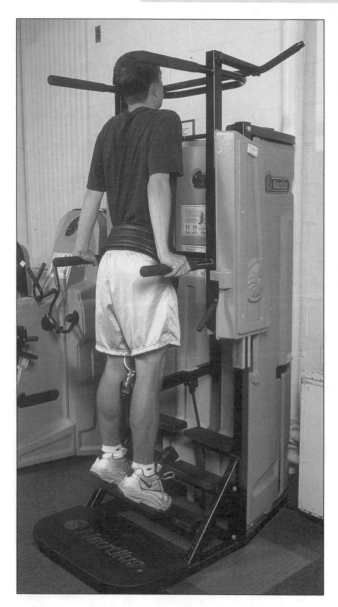

MUSCLES

- Gastrocnemius, soleus

PROCEDURE

- Place the belt securely around your waist; then stand with the balls of both feet on the edge of the step. Place your hands on the bar for support.
- Slowly lift your heels as high as possible while keeping your knees straight. Then return to the starting position, lowering your heels below step level.

Technique Tips

- Exhale as you lift the weight and inhale as you lower it.
- Wear appropriate footwear when performing this exercise.
- Maintain an erect posture with knees straight during this exercise.
- Do not bounce out of the bottom position.

Upper-Body Exercises

CHEST PRESS

MUSCLES

- Pectoralis major, anterior deltoid, triceps

PROCEDURE

- Position yourself so the handles are at chest level. Grasp the handles.
- Keep your head, shoulders, and back on the bench.
- Push the handles upward until you have almost extended, but not locked, your arms. Keep your wrists straight.
- Slowly return the handles to the starting position. Then begin the movement before the weight touches the stack.

Technique Tips

- Exhale during the lifting movement and inhale during the lowering movement.
- Do not lock your elbows in the extended position.
- Do not arch or twist your back when performing this exercise.

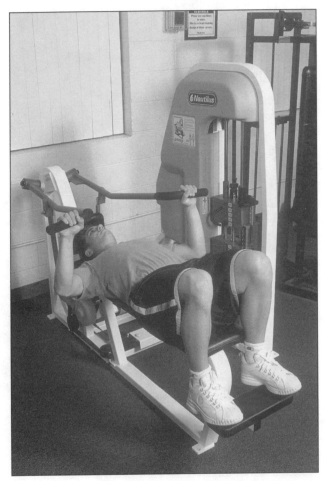

For Younger Athletes

- Grasp the handles at chest level.
- Stand erect and keep your back against the pad.
- Push handles forward until your arms are almost fully extended.
- Slowly return handles to starting position.

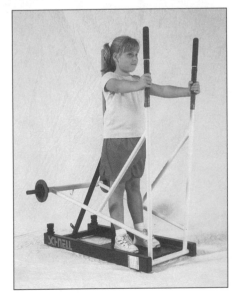

SEATED ROW

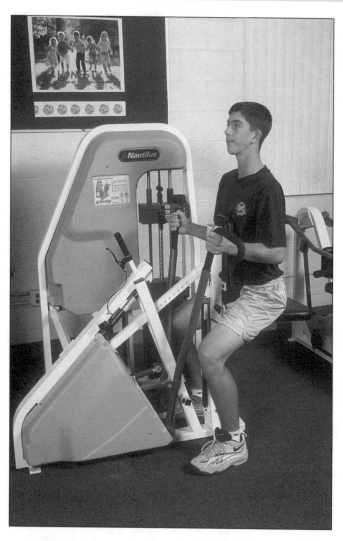

MUSCLES

- Latissimus dorsi, biceps

PROCEDURE

- Adjust the seat so the handles are at shoulder level. Sit with your chest against the pad, torso erect, and feet on the floor. Grasp both handles.
- Pull the handles back toward the side of your chest, keeping your chest on the pad.
- Slowly return the handles to the starting position. Then begin the movement before the weight touches the stack.

Technique Tips

- Exhale during the pulling movement and inhale during the return movement.
- Do not twist your back or allow your chest to come off the pad when performing this exercise.

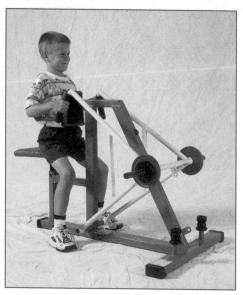

For Younger Athletes

- Grasp the handles with a firm, wrap-around grip.
- Keep chest against the pad throughout the entire pulling action.

FRONT PULLDOWN

MUSCLES

- Latissimus dorsi, biceps

PROCEDURE

- Grip the bar underhand (palms toward your face), about shoulder-width apart.
- Sit on the seat, placing both knees under the restraining pads, keeping your upper torso erect and arms straight.
- Slowly pull the bar downward below your chin. Then allow the bar to return slowly until you fully extend your arms.

Technique Tips

- Exhale during the pulling movement and inhale during the return movement.
- Do not twist your torso when performing this exercise. Use only your arms and upper back to complete the exercise.
- Keep the bar and cable away from your face during this exercise.

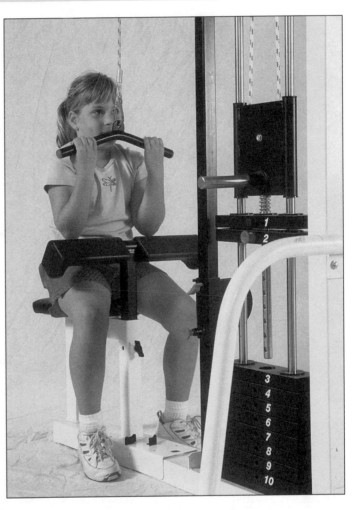

PULLOVER

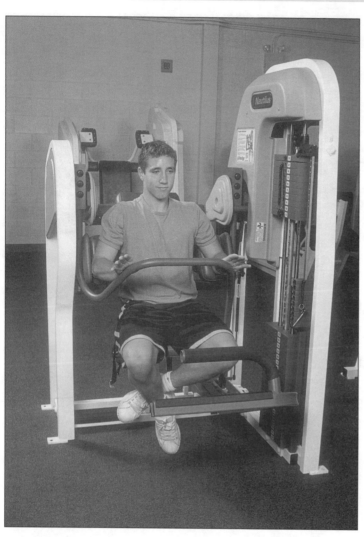

MUSCLES

- Latissimus dorsi

PROCEDURE

- Sit with your back against the pad and seat belt firmly secured with shoulder in line with the machine's axis of rotation. Press the foot lever forward and bring the arm pads into position.
- Position your elbows on the pads and place both hands on the bar. Slowly release the footpad, and allow your feet to hang in front of your body.
- Pull the arm pads downward until the bar touches your body. Slowly return to starting position and repeat.
- When finished, place your feet on the footpad, and press forward to hold the weight stack. Remove your arms and slowly lower the weight stack.

Technique Tips

- Exhale during the pulling movement and inhale during the return movement.
- Keep your hands open and elbows against the pad during this exercise.

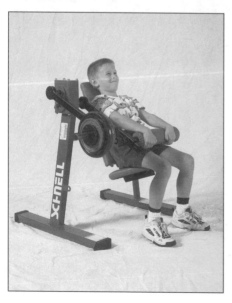

For Younger Athletes

- Adjust arm pad so that it contacts the wrist area.
- Keep back pressed firmly against the seat.
- Continue downward movement until arm pad touches the body.

OVERHEAD PRESS

MUSCLES

- Deltoids, triceps

PROCEDURE

- Adjust the seat so the handles are directly in front of the shoulders.
- Sit with your back against the pad and torso erect.
- Grasp the handles with a palms-forward grip about shoulder-width apart.
- Slowly push both arms overhead until you almost fully extend, but don't lock, your elbows.
- Slowly return to the starting position. Then begin the movement before the weight touches the stack.

Technique Tips

- Exhale during the lifting movement and inhale during the lowering movement.
- Keep your torso erect during this exercise.
- Learn this exercise with a light weight at first.

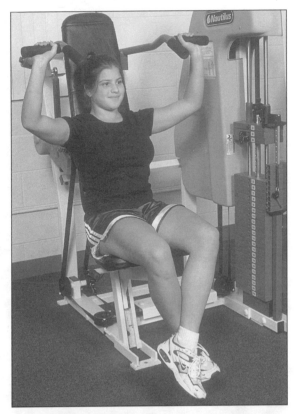

LATERAL RAISE

MUSCLES

- Deltoids

PROCEDURE

- Adjust the seat so the center of the shoulders are in line with the axis of rotation. Sit with your torso erect, and place your arms against the pads and your hands on the handles.
- Slowly lift both arms upward, keeping your wrists straight.
- Stop when your arms are parallel to the floor. Return to starting position.

Technique Tips

- Exhale as you lift the weight and inhale as you lower it.
- Stop the upward movement when your arms are parallel to the floor.
- Use your arms, not your hands, for lifting purposes.

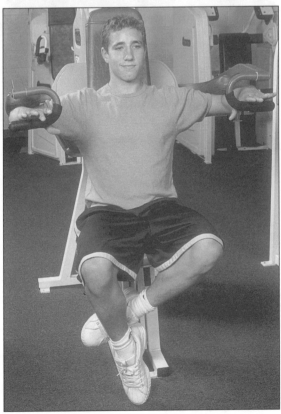

TRICEPS EXTENSION

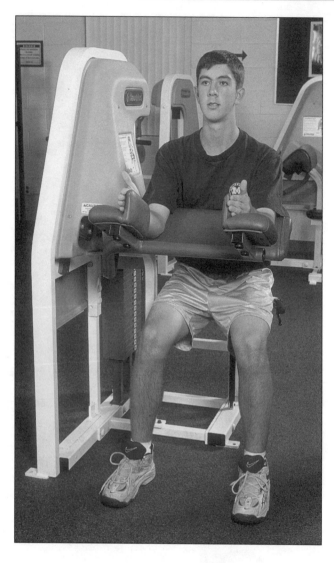

MUSCLES

- Triceps

PROCEDURE

- Adjust the seat so both elbows are in line with the machine's axis of rotation.
- Sit with your back against the pad, torso erect, and feet on the floor.
- Place the sides of your hands against the hand pads, and allow the pads to move close to your face.
- Slowly push both hand pads downward until you fully extend your arms. Then return to the starting position, beginning the movement before the weight touches the stack.

Technique Tips

- Exhale during the pushing movement and inhale during the return movement.
- Keep your upper arm on the pads and your wrists straight during this exercise.
- When finished, stand to remove your hands from the machine.

TRICEPS PRESSDOWN

MUSCLES

- Triceps

PROCEDURE

- Stand in front of the lat bar with your torso erect and knees slightly bent.
- Grasp the bar with both hands in an overhand grip (palms facing the floor), with your hands shoulder-width apart.
- Begin with the bar about shoulder level and your upper arms against your sides.
- Slowly press your forearms downward until you fully extend your arms.
- Then slowly return to the starting position, beginning the movement before the weight touches the stack.

Technique Tips

- Exhale during the pressing movement and inhale during the upward movement.
- Keep your torso erect, and do not allow your elbows to move forward or bow outward during this exercise.
- You can attach a short bar or other training accessories to the cable for this exercise.

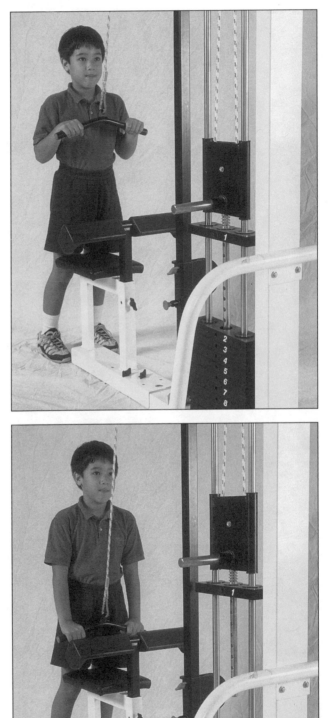

BICEPS CURL

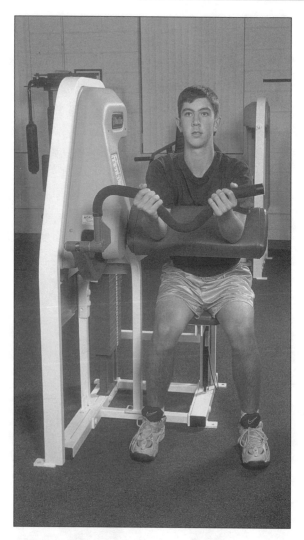

MUSCLES

- Biceps

PROCEDURE

- Adjust the seat so both elbows are in line with the machine's axis of rotation.
- Sit with your chest against the pad, torso erect, and feet on the floor.
- Grasp the handles with an underhand grip, elbows slightly bent.
- Slowly curl the handles upward until you fully flex your arms. Then return to the starting position, beginning the movement before the weight touches the stack.

Technique Tips

- Exhale during the curling movement and inhale during the lowering movement.
- Keep your upper arms on the pads and your wrists straight during this exercise.
- When finished, stand to remove your hands from the machine.

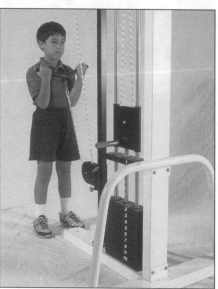

For Younger Athletes

- Stand straight and maintain an erect body position.
- Keep elbows firmly pressed against the sides.
- Only the forearms should move during the exercise.

ABDOMINAL CURL

MUSCLES

- Abdominals

PROCEDURE

- Adjust the seat so the navel is aligned with the machine's axis of rotation. Chest pads should be at chest level.
- Sit with your back against the pad, elbows on the pads, hands on the grips, and feet relaxed.
- Slowly curl your torso forward until you fully flex your trunk. Then return to the starting position, beginning the movement before the weight touches the stack.

Technique Tips

- Exhale during the curling movement and inhale during the return movement.
- Shorten the distance between the rib cage and the navel by contracting the abdominal muscles. Do not use your hands and shoulders.
- Avoid fast and jerky movements during this exercise.

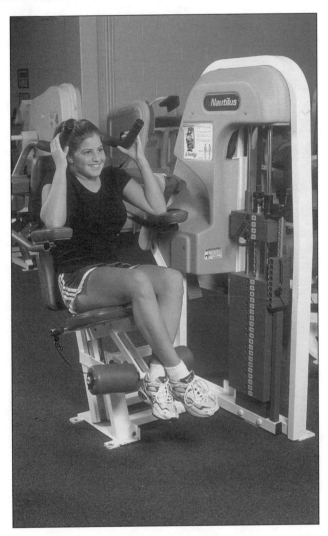

For Younger Athletes

- Chest pad should be below shoulders and secured with hands.
- Place feet on or under foot bar.

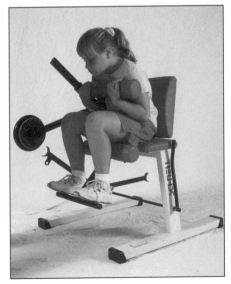

LOW-BACK EXTENSION

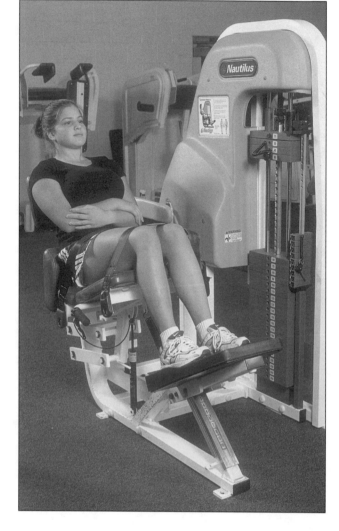

MUSCLES

- Erector spinae

PROCEDURE

- Adjust the seat so the navel is aligned with the machine's axis of rotation.
- Sit with your back against the pad, arms folded across your chest, and your feet firmly placed on the foot pad.
- Slowly extend your torso backward until you reach full trunk extension.

Technique Tips

- Exhale during the backward movement and inhale during the forward movement.
- Do not allow the upper body to free fall during the downward phase of this exercise.
- Avoid fast and jerky movements during this exercise.

ROTARY TORSO

MUSCLES

- Abdominals, external obliques, internal obliques

PROCEDURE

- Sit on the machine, facing forward with your legs around the seat extension.
- Place your left arm behind and your right arm against the movement pads.
- Slowly turn your torso to the right, and pause briefly; then return to the starting position, and perform the desired number of repetitions.
- Change the seat position and repeat to the left side.

Technique Tips

- Exhale as you lift the weight and inhale as you return to the starting position.
- Rotate your torso as far as possible, but stay within a pain-free range of motion.

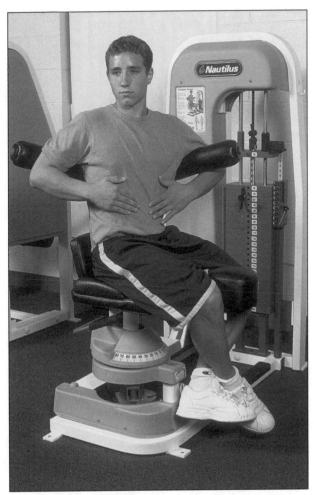

NECK FLEXION

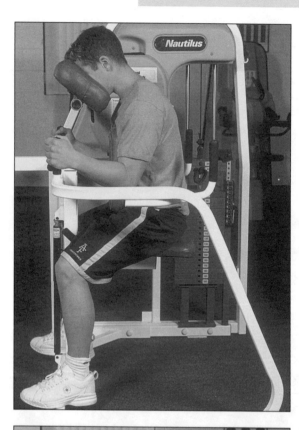

MUSCLES

- Neck flexors

PROCEDURE

- Adjust the seat and chest pad to the appropriate positions. Your face should fit in the face pad and your body should be erect.
- Place your forehead and cheeks against the face pad with your head angled slightly backward. Grasp the handles.
- Slowly push your head forward until your neck is comfortably flexed; then return to the starting position.

Technique Tips

- Exhale as you push your head forward and inhale on the return movement.
- Maintain chest contact with the pad during the exercise, and avoid fast or jerky movements.

NECK EXTENSION

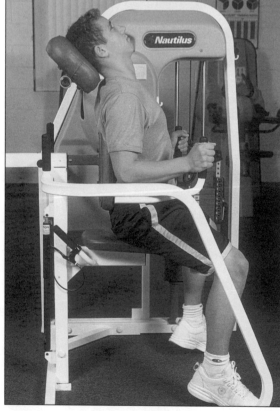

MUSCLES

- Neck extensors

PROCEDURE

- Adjust the seat and torso pad to the appropriate positions. The back of your head should fit in the head pad.
- Place the back of your head against the head pad with your head angled slightly forward. Grasp the handles.
- Slowly push your head backward until your neck is comfortably extended; then return to the starting position.

Technique Tips

- Exhale as you push the head backward and inhale on the return movement.
- Maintain torso contact with the pad during the exercise, and avoid fast or jerky movements.

SUPER FOREARM

MUSCLES

- Wrist flexors, wrist extensors, wrist supinators, wrist pronators, finger grippers

PROCEDURE

- This machine provides five separate exercises for the various muscles of the forearms. A qualified instructor should model each movement to demonstrate proper exercise execution.

Technique Tips

- Keep torso erect throughout each exercise.
- Keep forearms on restraining pads throughout each exercise.

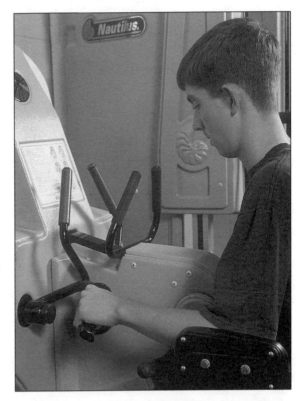

ROTARY SHOULDER

MUSCLES

- Shoulder rotator cuff, teres minor, infraspinatus, supraspinatus, subscapularis

PROCEDURE

- This machine provides four separate exercises for the internal and external rotator muscles of the shoulder. A qualified instructor should model each movement to demonstrate proper exercise execution.

Technique Tips

- Keep torso erect throughout each exercise.
- Keep elbow firmly secured in restraining cuff throughout each exercise.
- Use relatively light weight for the weaker internal rotation movements.

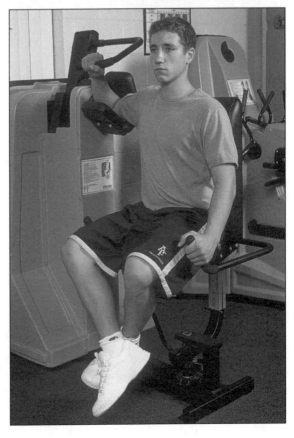

Summary

Weight machines are durable, versatile, safe, and easy to use. While most teenagers could probably fit into weight machines designed for adults, several companies have started to manufacture child-sized equipment that is designed to fit the smaller bodies of preadolescents. In either case, participants must fit into weight machines properly for safe and effective training. Also, it is important to remind participants to keep their hands and feet away from moving chains, pulleys and weight stacks. With proper instruction and supervision, children and teenagers can easily learn how to use different types of weight machines that train all of the major muscle groups. Machine training provides support, structure, and specific movement patterns that facilitate the learning process for a safe and effective exercise experience.

7

Cords and Balls

Rubber cords and medicine balls can be safe and effective alternatives to free weights and machines. Cords and balls are not only inexpensive and fun to use, but also add variety to a child's workout routine. Rubber cords and medicine balls come in different shapes and sizes, so children can start at safe levels and progress as needed. We use medicine balls and rubber cords in our youth fitness classes because several children can exercise simultaneously, and they can perform many different exercises. Further, you don't normally need spotting when performing medicine ball and rubber cord exercises, provided that you give appropriate guidance and instruction.

Strength training with a rubber cord involves performing exercises against the force required to stretch a rubber tube and return it to its unstretched state. Obviously, rubber cords must be made of elastic material that will stretch and provide resistance. Commercial rubber cord products are available from sporting good and fitness equipment stores, or you can make devices from a length of surgical tubing. You can perform exercises for the upper and lower body by either holding the ends of the cord with your hands or attaching the rubber cord to a fixed object. You can strengthen muscles by stretching the cord, which will provide resistance to the muscle or muscle group you want to strengthen. As children get stronger, you can increase the resistance by adjusting the amount of stretch on the cord or by using a thicker cord that will provide additional resistance.

Medicine balls are weighted vinyl, polyurethane, or leather balls that are available in different shapes and sizes. Although leather balls are popular, the drawback of this type of ball is that the stitching may fray and water may damage the outside covering. Adult athletes have used medicine ball exercises for many years, and now more children are benefiting from this mode of training. Unlike the traditional methods of strength training, medicine ball exercises condition the body through dynamic movements that you can perform either slowly or rapidly. Because you typically perform exercises on machines and free weights slowly (due to the nature of the equipment and the weight used), fast-speed medicine ball training can add a new dimension to a child's workout program. By using medicine balls of different weights and sizes, you can develop a conditioning program consisting of throwing and catching movements for the upper body, rotational exercises for the trunk, and extension exercises for the lower body. Most notably, you can use medicine balls to effectively strengthen the core of a child's body, which is where all movements begin. The core includes the abdominals as well as the hip and lower-back musculature. We have found that medicine ball training is a challenging, motivating, and worthwhile method of developing strength, speed, power, and coordination in children of all ages and abilities. In our programs we use color-coded balls and rubber cords so the instructors and the children can easily keep track of the loads they are using.

Training With Rubber Cords and Medicine Balls

Before you use tubes or balls, check that they are not torn or have abnormal wear and tear points. Do not use rubber cords that are torn or frayed for any exercise, because the cord could snap and cause an injury. Although most medicine balls can last for years, check the balls to be sure they are well made. Leather balls should be professionally stitched, and vinyl and polyurethane balls should be properly inflated. Again, it is worth emphasizing that rubber cords and medicine balls can be safe and effective for children, if adults provide competent instruction and supervision. Although rubber cords and medicine balls may seem harmless, they are not toys. Do not allow horseplay in the training area, and remind children that they can get hurt if they use the equipment improperly.

Strength-training exercises that use rubber tubing and medicine balls often require more skill and coordination than weight machines because children need to control the movement pattern. Therefore, adults need to provide clear instructions, and children should begin with a lightweight medicine ball or a thin rubber cord. Also note that the amount of stretch on the cord at the start of the exercise will affect the amount of resistance the child feels. When performing rubber cord exercises, adjust the child's hand position on the cord so he or she begins each exercise with an appropriate amount of stretch. In some cases it may be necessary to grasp a section of the tubing rather than the handles themselves. Depending on body size, limb length, and baseline strength level, a child's hand position on the cord will vary.

Rubber Cord Exercises

You can use the rubber cord exercises in this chapter to safely and effectively strengthen the upper and lower body. Remember that training with a rubber cord requires more skill and coordination than some other types of strength-training equipment. Beginning with a thin cord and focusing on the correct technique will give children an opportunity to learn how to stabilize their bodies when their arms or legs are working against the resistance of a rubber tube. When using rubber cords, note that the resistance from the cords will be greatest when the exercise motion nears completion. That is, unlike other types of strength-building equipment, the exercise will become more difficult at the end. Remind children that it is important to maintain proper form throughout the full range of motion.

RUBBER CORD SQUAT

MUSCLES

- Quadriceps, hamstrings, gluteals

PROCEDURE

- Begin by grasping the ends of a rubber cord in each hand, and stand erect with both feet on top of the middle of the cord to hold it stationary.
- Raise your hands to shoulder level with palms facing forward. The cords should be behind your shoulders.
- Slowly bend your ankles, knees, and hips until your thighs are parallel to the floor. Keep your back flat, head up, and eyes fixed straight ahead.
- Return to starting position by slowly straightening your knees and hips.

Technique Tips

- Your knees should follow a slightly outward pattern of the feet. Do not let the knees cave in.
- Inhale during the downward phase of the exercise and exhale during the upward phase.
- Avoid bouncing out of the bottom position.
- Concentrate on keeping your head up and chest out. Avoid excessive forward lean.

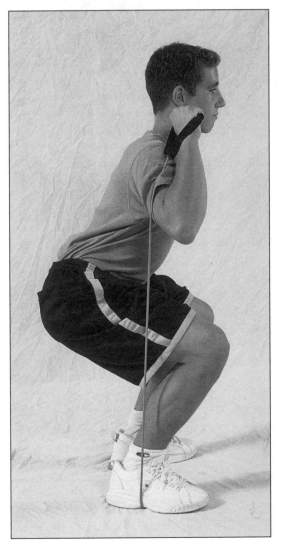

RUBBER CORD LEG CURL

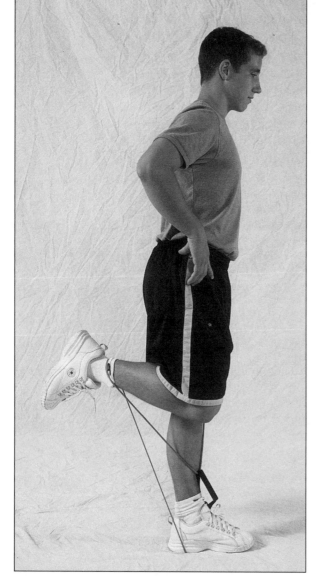

MUSCLES

- Hamstrings

PROCEDURE

- Put one handle of the cord through the opening near the other handle to create a small loop.
- Put your left foot inside the loop, and stand on the rubber cord. Put your right foot inside the loop, and place the cord behind your right ankle.
- Hold the rubber cord handle with your left hand and stand erect. Gently pull on the cord with your left hand until you feel a slight tension.
- Slowly curl your right leg backward toward your buttocks while maintaining an erect posture. Return your leg to the starting position, and perform the desired number of repetitions. Repeat on the other side.

Technique Tips

- Exhale during the lifting movement and inhale during the lowering movement.
- Keep the nonexercising leg stationary during this exercise.
- Use a thin cord at first.
- If necessary, place one hand on a wall or bench for balance.

RUBBER CORD STANDING CHEST PRESS

MUSCLES

- Pectoralis major, anterior deltoid, triceps

PROCEDURE

- Stand with your feet about shoulder-width apart and the rubber cord wrapped around the back of your shoulders.
- Grasp the ends of the cord firmly, and place both hands (palms facing the floor) in front of your shoulders with your elbows flexed.
- Slowly straighten your elbows until you fully extend both arms. Then return to the starting position and repeat.

Technique Tips

- Exhale during the pushing phase of the exercise and inhale during the return phase.
- Do not twist or arch your body.

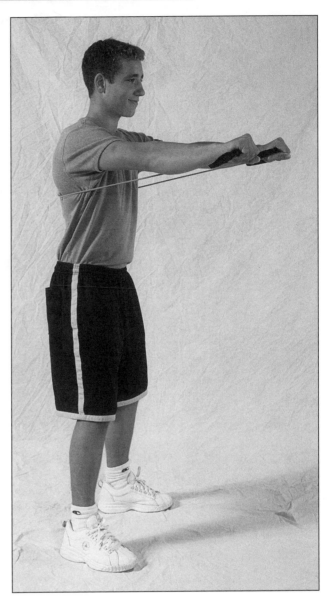

RUBBER CORD SEATED SHOULDER PRESS

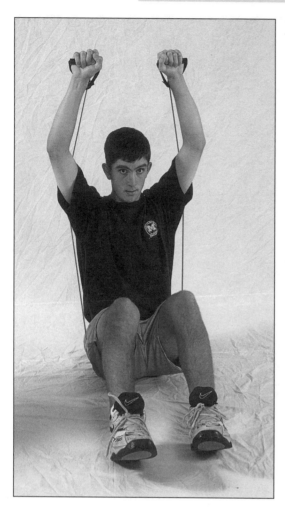

MUSCLES

- Deltoids, upper trapezius, triceps

PROCEDURE

- Begin by sitting on the middle of a rubber cord while holding an end of the cord in each hand.
- Hold the cord at shoulder height with your palms facing away from your body.
- Slowly push both arms upward until you fully extend them over the shoulders. Then lower your arms to the starting position and repeat.

Technique Tips

- Exhale during the lifting phase of the exercise and inhale during the lowering phase.
- Sit erect and keep your lower back straight by contracting your abdominal and lower-back muscles.

RUBBER CORD UPRIGHT ROW

MUSCLES

- Deltoids, upper trapezius, biceps

PROCEDURE

- Begin by grasping one end of the cord in each hand and standing erect with both feet on top of the cord about hip-width apart. Hold the cord so it hangs straight down in front of your body with your palms facing your body. The hands should be closer than shoulder-width apart.
- Slowly pull both hands upward to the height of the upper chest; then lower them to the starting position.

Technique Tips

- Exhale during the lifting phase of the exercise and inhale during the lowering phase.
- Stand erect and keep the cord close to your body during this exercise.
- At the top of the movement the elbows should be higher than the shoulders.

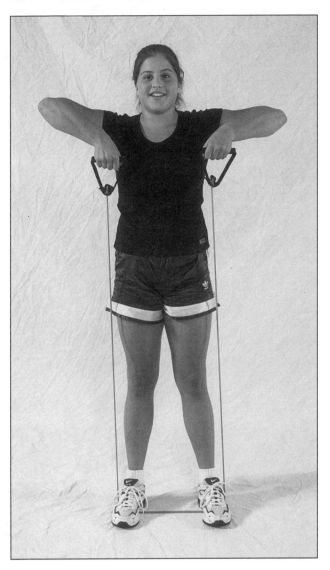

RUBBER CORD LATERAL RAISE

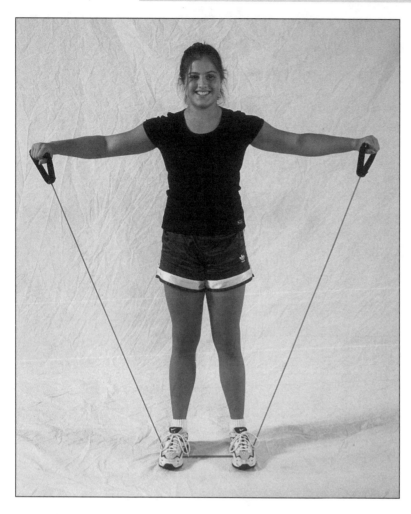

MUSCLES

- Deltoids

PROCEDURE

- Begin by grasping one end of the cord in each hand and standing erect with both feet on top of the cord about hip-width apart. Hold the cord so it hangs straight down at your sides with your palms facing your body and elbows slightly bent.
- Slowly lift both arms upward and sideward until your arms are level with your shoulders (arms parallel to floor). Keep elbows slightly bent and return to starting position.

Technique Tips

- Exhale during the lifting phase of the exercise and inhale during the lowering phase.
- Stand erect and keep your lower back straight by contracting your abdominal and lower-back muscles.
- Don't raise your arms higher than parallel to the floor.

RUBBER CORD LAT PULLDOWN

MUSCLES

- Latissimus dorsi, biceps

PROCEDURE

- Grip a section of the cord with your hands about shoulder-width apart, and fully extend your arms overhead. Stand erect with your hands wider than your shoulders and your palms facing forward.
- Slowly pull your arms downward until the cord is behind your neck and your arms are parallel to the floor. Then return slowly to starting position.

Technique Tips

- Exhale during the downward movement and inhale during the return movement.
- Use only your arms and upper back to complete the exercise. Focus on pulling your shoulder blades together and keeping your arms in line with your body.
- Fold the cord in half for greater resistance.

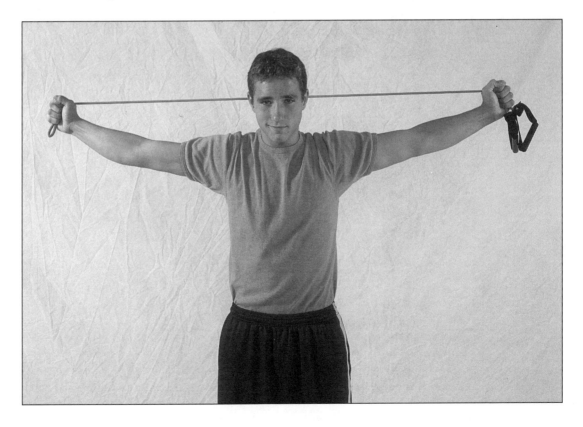

RUBBER CORD SEATED ROW

MUSCLES

- Latissimus dorsi, biceps

PROCEDURE

- Begin by wrapping the cord around your feet. Grasp the handles of the cord. Sit on the floor with your knees slightly bent, your back straight, and your palms facing each other.
- Pull the cord handles back toward the sides of your body; then slowly return the handles to the starting position.

Technique Tips

- Exhale during the pulling movement and inhale during the return movement.
- Check to be sure the rubber cord is securely wrapped around your feet. Point your toes forward slightly to prevent the cord from slipping off your feet.
- As an alternative, you can place the rubber cord around an immovable object while in the seated position.

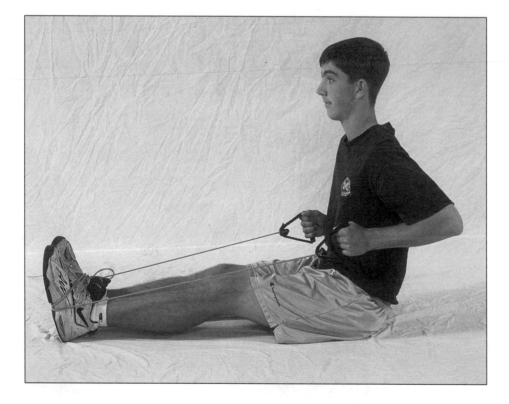

RUBBER CORD BICEPS CURL

MUSCLES

- Biceps

PROCEDURE

- Begin by standing on top of the cord with your body erect and both hands grasping the cord handles. Place your feet about hip-width apart, and fully extend your arms with your palms facing forward.
- Slowly curl both hands upward toward your shoulders until your palms face the chest. Then lower both arms to the starting position.

Technique Tips

- Exhale during the lifting phase of the exercise and inhale during the lowering phase.
- Stand erect and keep your lower back straight by contracting your abdominal and lower-back muscles.
- If necessary, stand with your back against the wall to prevent upper-body torso movement.
- Do not step off the cord unless your arms are in the starting position.

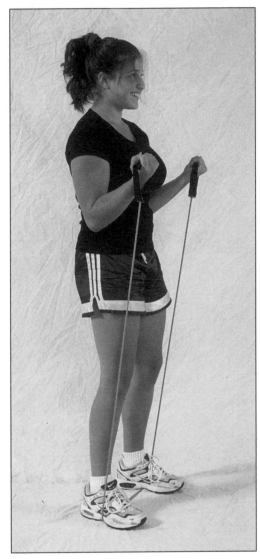

RUBBER CORD TRICEPS EXTENSION

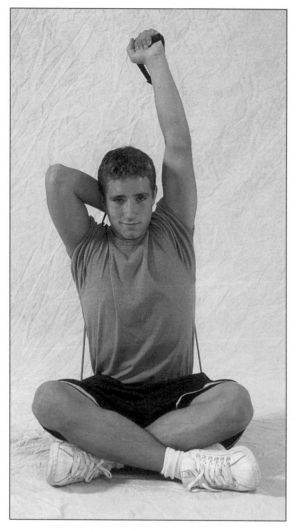

MUSCLES

- Triceps

PROCEDURE

- Begin by sitting on the middle of a rubber cord while holding an end of the cord in each hand.
- Place both hands behind your head with your palms facing the ceiling. The elbows should be bent.
- Slowly push one arm upward until you fully extend it over your head. Then lower your arm to the starting position, and repeat with your other arm.

Technique Tips

- Exhale during the pushing phase of the exercise and inhale during the lowering phase.
- Only the elbow and forearm should move during this exercise.
- Be sure you secure the cord beneath your buttocks.

Medicine Ball Exercises

You can control the intensity of a medicine ball exercise by the weight of the medicine ball and the speed at which you perform the exercise. In our program we begin with one-kilogram medicine balls and teach children how to perform the basic exercises properly. Once children have mastered the proper form, we gradually increase the speed of some exercise movements, the weight of the medicine ball (by about one-half kilogram at a time), and, when appropriate, the distance between training partners. By gradually increasing the speed of movement and the weight of the ball, you can use this type of training to enhance the strength and speed of muscle action.

It is desirable to have medicine balls of different weights and sizes on hand to accommodate the needs and abilities of all children. Also, you will need lighter balls for one-arm exercises and heavier balls for two-arm exercises. We organized the medicine ball exercises into three sections: warm-up, strength, and power exercises. We note the specific muscles used for the strength exercises, whereas we identify general

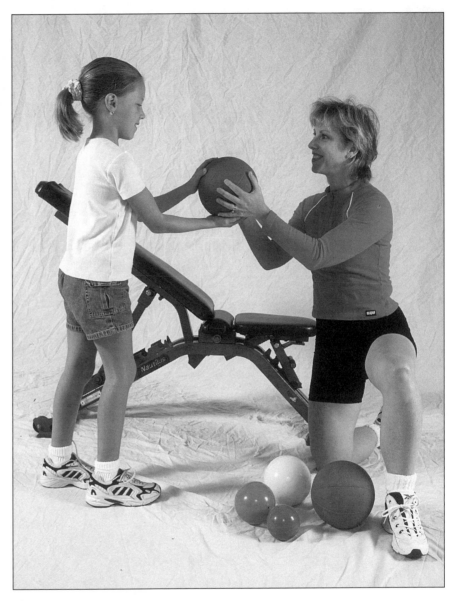

Medicine balls come in a variety of weights and sizes.

body parts for the power exercises. Just as for other modes of training, you should perform warm-up and strength exercises with medicine balls in a slow and controlled manner; however, you can perform power exercises at a faster speed provided that you maintain proper form. Before performing power exercises, always do a few warm-up repetitions of the same exercise at a slow speed. In our program children perform the power exercises with medicine balls before strength exercises, because if they are fatigued before performing the power exercises they will have difficulty generating near-maximal power, which is the goal of the exercise.

Warm-Up Exercises

The following five exercises are warm-ups for the entire body and therefore specific muscle groups are not mentioned.

AROUND THE WORLD

PROCEDURE

- Stand with your feet about shoulder-width apart, and hold a light medicine ball over your head with your arms fully extended.
- Move the ball in a giant circle, bending your knees as the ball moves to the bottom of the circle and straightening your knees as the ball moves to the top of the circle. Complete the desired number of repetitions; then move the ball in the opposite direction.

BALL MARCH

PROCEDURE

- Stand with your feet about shoulder-width apart, and hold a light medicine ball in front of your body at chest height.
- As you lift one knee to waist level, touch the ball to the knee; then return the ball and knee to starting position. Repeat with opposite leg.

JOG AND CATCH

PROCEDURE

- Stand with your feet about shoulder-width apart, and hold a light medicine ball in front of your body at waist height.
- Jog in place while playing catch with the ball. For variety, children can clap their hands while the ball is in the air.

BODY STRETCH

PROCEDURE

- Stand with your feet about shoulder-width apart, and hold a light medicine ball in front of your body at chest height.
- Extend your arms overhead, reaching toward one side of your body. Return to starting position and repeat to the opposite side.

HELICOPTER CIRCLES

PROCEDURE

- Sit on the floor with your legs extended in front of your body and slightly apart.
- Hold the medicine ball over your head with your arms extended. Move the ball in large circles overhead without losing your balance.

Strength Exercises

FRONT SQUAT

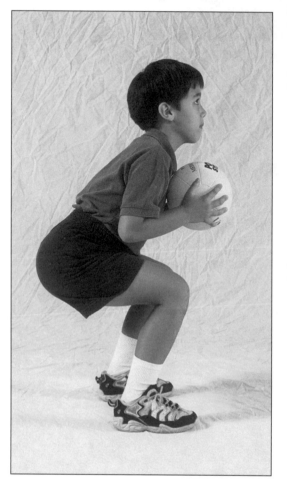

MUSCLES

- Quadriceps, hamstrings, gluteals

PROCEDURE

- Begin by holding a medicine ball directly in front of your chest with your feet about hip-width apart and toes pointing slightly outward.
- Slowly bend your ankles, knees, and hips until your thighs are parallel to the floor. Keep your back flat, head up, and eyes fixed straight ahead.
- Return to the starting position by slowly straightening your knees and hips.

Technique Tips

- Your knees should follow a slightly outward pattern of the feet. Do not let the knees cave in.
- Inhale during the downward phase of the exercise and exhale during the upward phase.
- Avoid bouncing out of the bottom position.
- Concentrate on keeping your head up and chest out. Avoid excessive forward lean.
- For variety, you can perform an overhead squat by holding a medicine ball overhead with your arms fully extended. Follow procedures as noted previously, keeping your arms extended during the exercise.

FRONT SHOULDER RAISE

MUSCLES

- Deltoids

PROCEDURE

- Begin by holding a medicine ball in front of your waist with both hands. Stand erect with your feet about hip-width apart.
- Slowly lift the ball upward until your arms are at shoulder height; then return to the starting position and repeat.

Technique Tips

- Exhale during the lifting phase of the exercise and inhale during the lowering phase.
- Stand erect and keep your lower back straight by contracting your abdominal and lower-back muscles.
- Don't raise your arms higher than parallel to the floor.

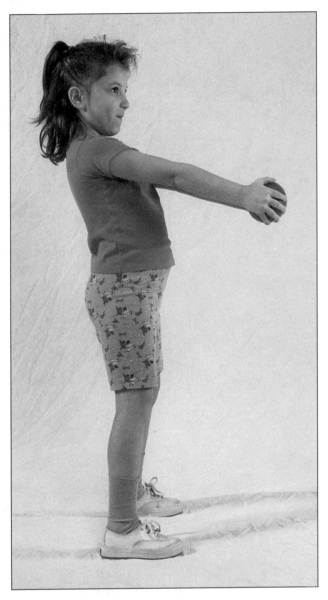

SUPINE CHEST PRESS

MUSCLES

- Pectoralis major, anterior deltoid, triceps

PROCEDURE

- Lie on your back holding a medicine ball on your chest.
- Slowly press the ball off your chest until you fully extend both arms. Then slowly return to starting position.

Technique Tips

- Exhale during the pressing phase of the exercise and inhale during the lowering phase.
- Keep the ball above your chest, not above your face.

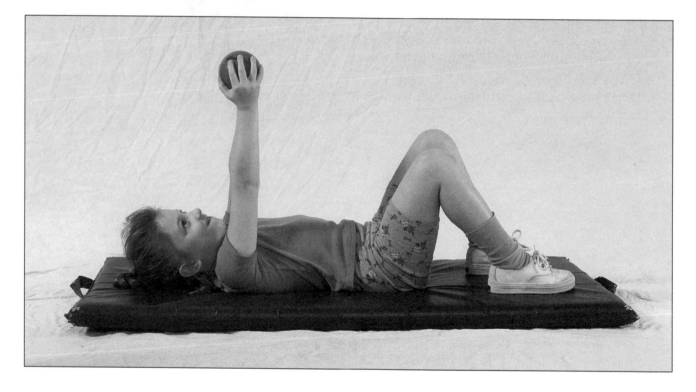

TRICEPS PRESS

MUSCLES

- Triceps

PROCEDURE

- Stand erect with your feet about hip-width apart. Hold a medicine ball behind your head with your elbows flexed at ear level.
- Press the ball overhead until you fully extend your arms. Then slowly return to starting position and repeat.

Technique Tips

- Exhale during the lifting phase of the exercise and inhale during the lowering phase.
- Stand erect and keep your lower back straight by contracting your abdominal and lower-back muscles.
- Only the elbows and forearms should move during this exercise.

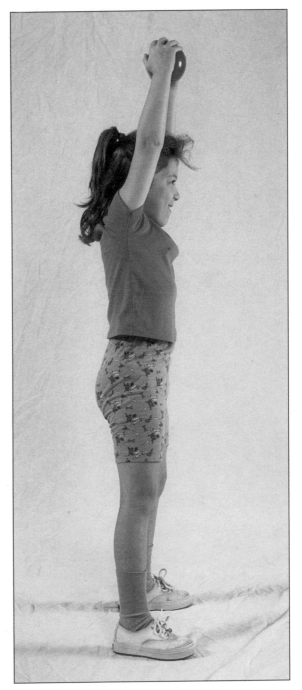

BICEPS CURL

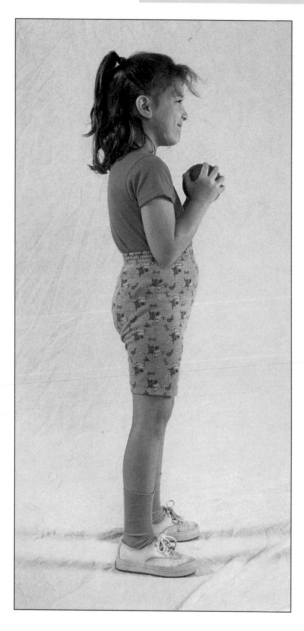

MUSCLES

- Biceps

PROCEDURE

- Stand erect with your feet about hip-width apart. Hold a medicine ball in front of your waist with your arms fully extended.
- Curl the ball toward your face, keeping your back straight. Then slowly return to starting position and repeat.

Technique Tips

- Exhale during the curling phase of the exercise and inhale during the lowering phase.
- Stand erect and keep your lower back straight by contracting your abdominal and lower-back muscles.
- Only the elbows and forearms should move during this exercise.

TWIST AND TURN

MUSCLES

- Abdominals, obliques

PROCEDURE

- Sit on the floor with your knees bent at a 45-degree angle and your feet on the floor. Hold a medicine ball in front of your body with your arms extended.
- Rotate your upper body from side-to-side, touching the floor with the ball on each side.

Technique Tips

- Lean back slightly while rotating your body from side-to-side.
- For variety, perform a partner twist by having two children sit or stand back-to-back. They pass the ball to each other in a circle for a desired number of repetitions; then change the direction.

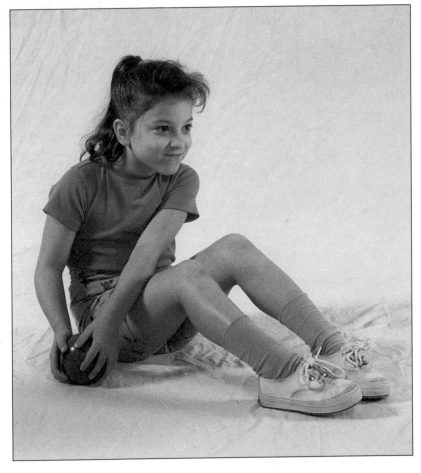

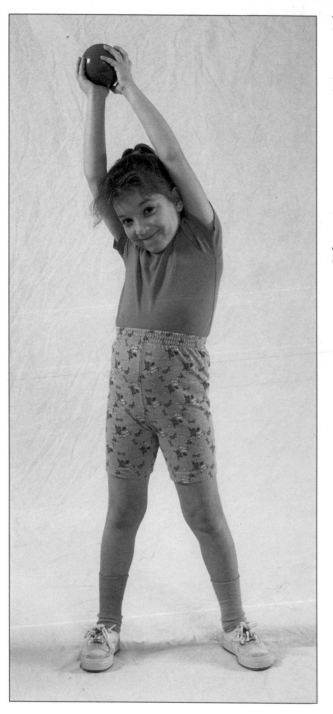

SIDE BEND

MUSCLES

- Abdominals, obliques

PROCEDURE

- Stand erect with your feet about hip-width apart and your knees slightly bent. Hold a medicine ball overhead with your arms fully extended.
- Slowly bend to one side, keeping your back and arms straight. Return to starting position and repeat to the other side.

Technique Tips

- Exhale during the lowering phase of the exercise and inhale during the upward phase.
- Move only from side-to-side. Avoid leaning forward.

Power Exercises

SQUAT TOSS

MUSCLES

- Legs, chest, arms

PROCEDURE

- Begin by holding a medicine ball directly in front of your chest with your feet about hip-width apart and toes pointing slightly outward.
- Slowly bend your ankles, knees, and hips until your thighs are parallel to the floor. Keep your back flat, head up, and eyes fixed straight ahead.
- Quickly jump upward and toss the ball as high as you can in front of you.

Technique Tips

- On the downward motion, your knees should follow a slightly outward pattern of the feet. Do not let the knees cave in.
- Inhale during the downward phase of the exercise and exhale during the upward phase.
- Avoid bouncing out of the bottom position.

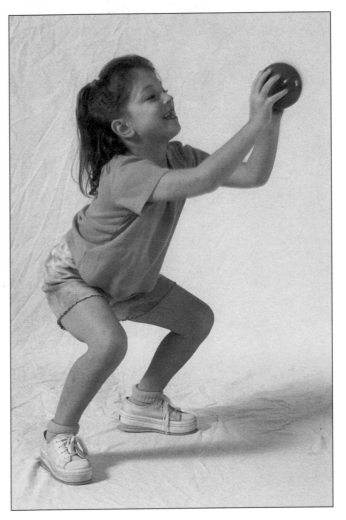

LUNGE PASS

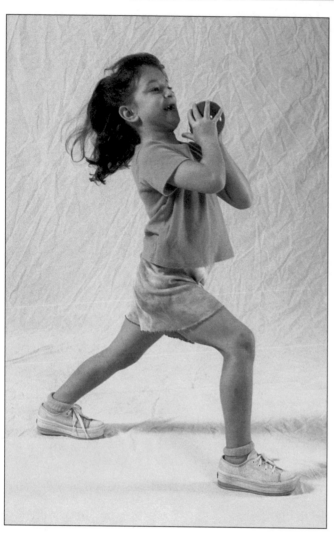

MUSCLES

- Legs, chest, arms

PROCEDURE

- Begin by holding a medicine ball directly in front of your chest with feet about hip-width apart.
- Take a long step forward, and quickly push the ball off your chest.

Technique Tips

- Exhale as you push the ball off your chest.
- Keep your upper torso erect after your release the ball. Do not lean forward.
- Step far enough in front of your body so your front knee is bent to nearly 90 degrees.

CHEST PASS

MUSCLES

- Chest, arms

PROCEDURE

- Stand erect while holding a medicine ball at chest level with both hands.
- Step forward and press the ball off your chest.

Technique Tips

- Exhale as you push the ball off your chest.
- Keep your upper torso erect after you release the ball. Do not lean forward.
- A partner can stand about 10 feet away and catch the ball. Over time the children can increase the distance between partners. The farther the distance, the greater the effort that is required.
- For variety, you can perform this exercise while kneeling on the floor. Keep your body straight as you push the ball off your chest.

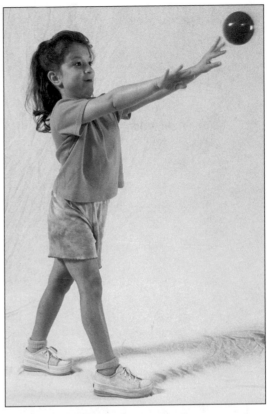

SIDE PASS

MUSCLES

- Trunk, arms

PROCEDURE

- Stand with your side facing your partner. With the ball about waist level, swing it across your body and pass it to your partner. When you have performed the desired number of repetitions, stand with the other side of your body facing your partner and repeat.

Technique Tips

- Exhale as you throw the ball to your partner.
- Do not move your feet during this exercise. Move only your arms and trunk.

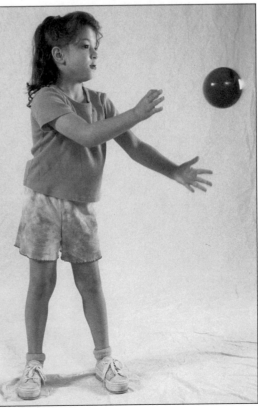

UNDERHAND THROW

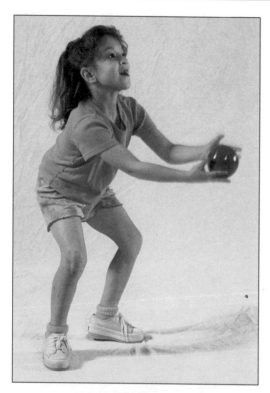

MUSCLES

- Legs, shoulders, trunk, arms

PROCEDURE

- Hold the medicine ball in a squat position with your arms straight and the ball close to the floor.
- Come up from the squat position, and throw the ball as far as you can.

Technique Tips

- Exhale as you throw the ball.
- Lift your body straight up, and keep your back erect.

SINGLE-ARM THROW

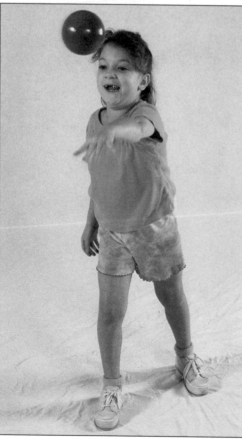

MUSCLES

- Trunk, arms

PROCEDURE

- Hold a small medicine ball in one hand at ear level.
- Step forward and throw the ball as far as you can with standard throwing action. Repeat with your other arm.

Technique Tips

- Because you use only one arm, begin with a lightweight medicine ball and gradually progress as you get stronger.
- For variety, you can perform this exercise while kneeling on the floor.

Summary

Cords and balls are not only inexpensive and easy to use, but they can add a new dimension to a child's workout routine. Rubber cords are made of elastic material that can provide a challenging resistance to the muscle or muscle groups you want to strengthen. Adults have used medicine balls for many years, and now they are available in a variety of shapes and sizes that are appropriate for children. Unlike other methods of conditioning, medicine ball training involves dynamic movements that can be performed either slowly or rapidly. Medicine ball training can be a safe and challenging method of developing strength, power, balance, and coordination in children and teenagers of all abilities. Since strength training with cords and balls involves skill and coordination, we take the time to provide clear instructions and begin with a thin rubber cord or a lightweight medicine ball.

Body-Weight Exercises

Body-weight exercises are one of the oldest forms of strength training. This type of exercise simply involves using your body weight as resistance. Push-ups, pull-ups, and sit-ups are examples of body-weight exercises that you can use to develop muscle strength and muscle endurance. Obviously, a major advantage of body-weight training is that you need no equipment, and therefore the cost is free. Also, you can perform a variety of exercises, and many children can strength train at the same time. One drawback of body-weight training is the difficulty in adjusting the body weight to the strength level. Some children may not be strong enough to perform even one repetition of an exercise, whereas other children may be able to perform 30 repetitions or more.

Like other types of strength training, body-weight training can be a safe and effective method of conditioning, provided that children learn how to perform the exercises correctly. In our programs we want children to experience success while strength training, so we carefully choose the body-weight exercises that are appropriate for each child's strength level. For example, if we are working with a group of overweight children who have never strength trained before, we may use only one or two body-weight exercises for the legs and abdominals and use

121

adjustable weights for upper-body conditioning. Asking an out of shape child to attempt one pull-up in front of his or her friends is not only an ineffective method of strength training, but also a potentially humiliating experience.

Once children develop enough strength to handle their body weight, it is possible to develop a total-body workout using body-weight exercises. We have found body-weight circuit training to be a safe, effective, and inexpensive method of training for young athletes. In this method of training, children move from one body-weight exercise to the next with about a minute of rest between exercises. However, this type of training can be aerobically taxing, and therefore, you should gradually increase the volume and intensity of training. That is, give children an opportunity to learn new exercises and adapt to the demands of the training stimulus before the program becomes too challenging and unpleasant. Over time, you can add exercises and reduce the rest period between exercises.

Body-Weight Training

The principles of performing body-weight exercises are the same as other strength-training methods. Children should warm up before they strength train and should always wear appropriate attire (including athletic shoes). Children should perform exercises in a controlled manner throughout the full range of motion and should breath continuously during the exercise. It makes sense to begin with exercises that are less demanding and progress to exercises that are more challenging as strength increases. In some cases, it may be necessary to modify a traditional exercise to make it easier to perform. For example, performing a push-up from the knees or against a wall may be appropriate for some children who find the standard push-up too difficult. The modified versions work the same muscle groups but require lifting less weight.

Body-Weight Exercises

You can use body-weight exercises to safely and effectively strengthen all the major muscle groups. Many different body-weight exercises are possible. It is desirable to begin with exercises that you can comfortably perform for the desired number of repetitions and gradually increase the difficulty of the exercise over time. We have organized the body-weight exercises into three sections: lower body, upper body, and midsection.

Lower-Body Exercises

SQUAT

MUSCLES

- Quadriceps, hamstrings, gluteals

PROCEDURE

- Begin by standing erect with your feet about hip-width apart and toes pointing slightly outward. Place your hands on your hips or straight out in front of your body.
- Slowly bend your ankles, knees, and hips until your thighs are parallel to the floor. Keep your back flat, head up, and eyes fixed straight ahead. Pause briefly in the bottom position.
- Return to starting position by slowly straightening your knees and hips.

Technique Tips

- Inhale during the downward phase of the exercise and exhale during the upward phase.
- Your knees should follow a slightly outward pattern of the feet. Do not let the knees cave in.
- Avoid bouncing out of the bottom position.
- Concentrate on keeping your head up and chest out. Avoid excessive forward lean.

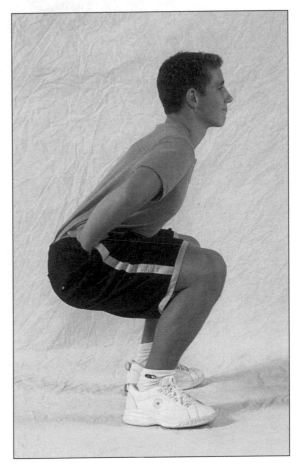

WALKING LUNGE

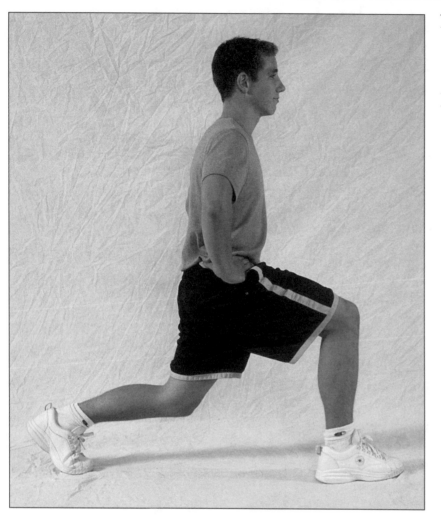

MUSCLES

- Quadriceps, hamstrings, gluteals

PROCEDURE

- Begin by standing erect with your feet about hip-width apart. Hold your arms at your sides and look straight forward.

- Take a long step forward with your right leg; bend the knee of the right leg and lower your body. The thigh of the right leg should be parallel to the floor, and the right knee should be over the ankle of the right foot. Bend the left knee slightly.

- Then lift your body upward slightly, and step forward with your left leg. Bring your left leg forward, and lower your body until the thigh of your left leg is parallel to the floor. Continue to walk forward alternating legs.

Technique Tips

- Keep your head up, back upright, and shoulders over the hips.
- This exercise requires balance and coordination. Take your time to learn the proper form.
- Avoid using upper-torso momentum to return to the starting position. Concentrate on keeping your back upright throughout the exercise.

HEEL RAISE

MUSCLES

- Gastrocnemius, soleus

PROCEDURE

- Begin by standing erect with your feet about hip-width apart. Place the full ball of the right foot on a board or step with the heel off the surface. Use the free left hand for balance by holding onto the wall or banister. Wrap the left foot around the right ankle.

- Rise onto the right toe as high as possible with right knee straight; then slowly lower the heel as far as comfortable. Complete the assigned number of repetitions, and repeat with opposite leg.

Technique Tips

- Inhale during the lowering phase of the exercise and exhale during the upward phase.

- Concentrate on keeping your torso and knees straight to avoid upper-leg involvement.

- If this exercise is too difficult, you can perform it with both feet on a board or step.

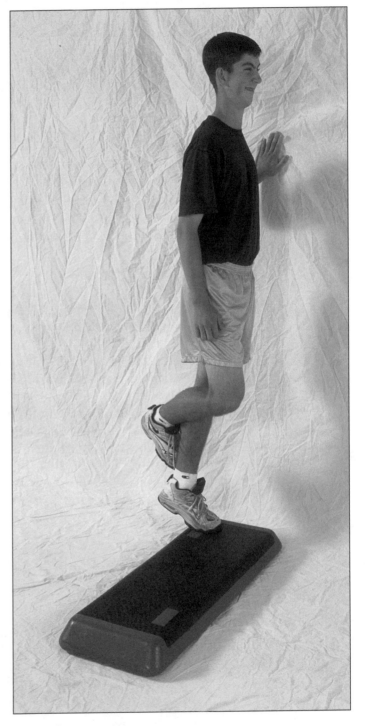

Upper-Body Exercises

PUSH-UP

MUSCLES

- Pectoralis major, deltoids, triceps

PROCEDURE

- Lie face down on the floor with your body straight, legs slightly apart, and hands slightly more than shoulder-width apart facing forward. Lift your body on your hands and toes.
- While keeping your back flat, slowly lower your body by bending your elbows until your chest touches the floor. Pause briefly, then push away from the floor until you fully extend your arms.

Technique Tips

- Inhale as you lower your body and exhale as you press your body upward.
- Keep the back and legs straight throughout this exercise.

If this exercise is too difficult, try a wall push-up or a bent-knee push-up. To perform a wall push-up, stand about two feet from a wall and place your hands slightly wider than shoulder-width apart on the wall. Slowly lower your body close to the wall, pause briefly, then return to starting position. To perform a bent-knee push-up, lie face down on the floor with your body straight and hands slightly wider than shoulder-width apart. Bend your knees and keep your feet close together. The weight of your body should be on your hands and knees. Support your body with your arms fully extended. Slowly lower your body by bending your elbows until your chest touches the floor. Pause briefly, then push away from the floor until you fully extend your arms.

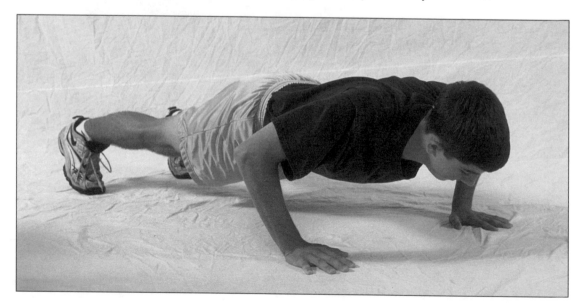

CHIN-UP

MUSCLES

- Latissimus dorsi, biceps

PROCEDURE

- Grasp a bar overhead with arms extended and torso straight. Hands should be about shoulder-width apart and palms should face your body.
- Pull your body upward until your chin is above the bar; then lower your body to the starting position.

Technique Tips

- Exhale as you pull your body upward and inhale as you lower it.
- If you need assistance with this exercise, a spotter can help by placing his or her hands on your waist and lifting your body upward.
- Be careful when letting go of the bar. If necessary, an adult spotter should provide assistance.
- For variety, try a wide-grip pull-up with your palms facing away from your body.
- For some children, chin-ups and pull-ups may be too difficult. In this case, begin with a front pulldown on a weight machine or a chin-up on a weight-assisted chin-dip machine.
- This technique may also be performed on a weight-assisted machine that reduces body weight by a counterweight system.

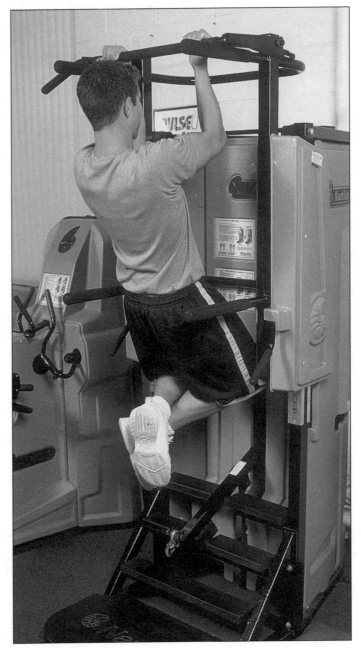

BAR DIP

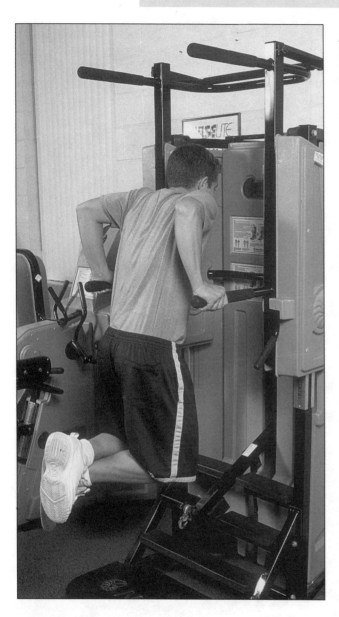

MUSCLES

- Triceps, pectoralis major, deltoids

PROCEDURE

- Grip the dip bar with palms facing each other and arms fully extended. Keep your body straight.
- Slowly lower your body until the elbows are at right angles. Then push upward to the starting position.

Technique Tips

- Inhale as you lower your body and exhale as you press your body upward.
- Avoid swinging your body during this exercise, and do not bounce out of the bottom position.
- If your feet touch the floor, cross your lower legs.
- This exercise may also be performed on a weight-assisted machine that reduces body weight by a counterweight system.

If you cannot complete a dip with the proper technique, use a weight-assisted chin-dip machine with an adjustable weight stack or a chair dip. To perform a chair dip, place the heels of your hand about shoulder-width apart on the front edge of a chair or bench. Fully extend your elbows so your arms are straight. Your fingers should point toward your body, and your legs should be straight, with both feet on the floor. Slowly lower your body until your elbows form right angles. Then return to the starting position. Make sure the chair or bench is secure so it will not slip during this exercise.

Midsection Exercises

TRUNK CURL AND DIAGONAL TRUNK CURL

MUSCLES

- Abdominals

PROCEDURE

- Lie on the floor with your knees bent and feet on the floor. Place your hands on your thighs with your arms fully extended.

- Slowly curl your shoulders and upper back off the floor while sliding your hands up your thighs. Keep your lower back on the floor. Your hands should reach your kneecaps.

- Pause momentarily, then return to the starting position.

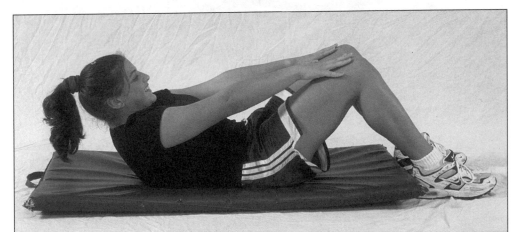

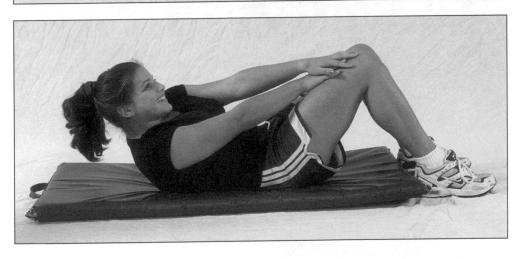

Technique Tips

- Exhale as you curl your body upward and inhale as you lower your body.
- You can place both hands across your chest or behind your head during this exercise. However, if you place your hands behind your head, be careful not to pull your head forward with your hands during the exercise.

For variety, you can try a diagonal trunk curl, which emphasizes the obliques on the sides of the midsection. Assume the same starting position with your arms extended in front of your body. Reach your left hand toward your right kneecap, and slowly return to starting position; then reach your right hand toward your left kneecap. Your lower back should remain in contact with the floor during this exercise.

HANGING-KNEE RAISE

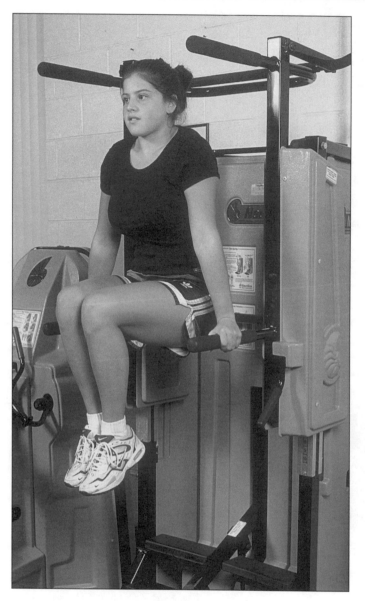

MUSCLES

- Abdominals, hip flexors

PROCEDURE

- Grasp the dip bars with both hands, and let your body hang with your arms fully extended. If available, use a knee-raise unit, position your forearms on the pads, and place your back against the support.
- Begin the movement by lifting your bent knees toward your chest. Pause briefly, then lower the legs to the starting position.

Technique Tips

- Exhale as you lift your legs and inhale as you lower them.
- Keep your back and arms motionless during this exercise. If needed, a spotter can place his or her hand on your lower back to prevent swinging or jerking motions.

PELVIC TILT

MUSCLES

- Abdominals

PROCEDURE

- Lie on the floor with your knees bent and feet on the floor. Place your hands loosely behind your head.
- Slowly press your lower back against the floor by tightening your abdominals. Hold this position for five seconds; then return to the starting position.

Technique Tips

- Exhale as you press your lower back into the floor and inhale as you return to the starting position.

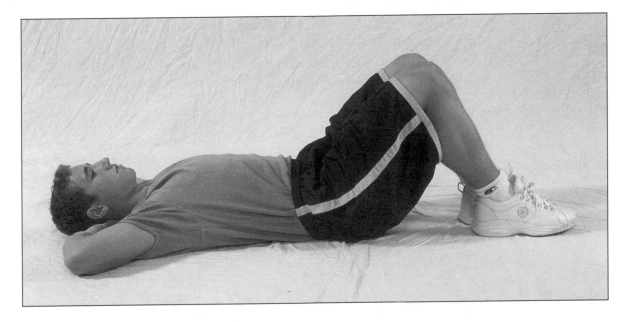

KNEELING-TRUNK EXTENSION

MUSCLES

- Spinal erectors

PROCEDURE

- Kneel on the floor, supporting your body on both hands and both knees.
- Slowly extend your right leg backward until it is parallel to the floor. Pause momentarily, then return your right leg to the starting position and extend your left leg backward. Pause momentarily, then return your left leg to the starting position and continue to alternate legs.

Technique Tips

- Exhale as you extend your leg backward and inhale as you return your leg to the starting position.
- Perform this exercise in a slow and controlled manner. Do not raise your limbs higher than parallel to the floor.
- For a more challenging exercise, raise your left arm parallel to the floor while you extend your right leg (and vice versa).

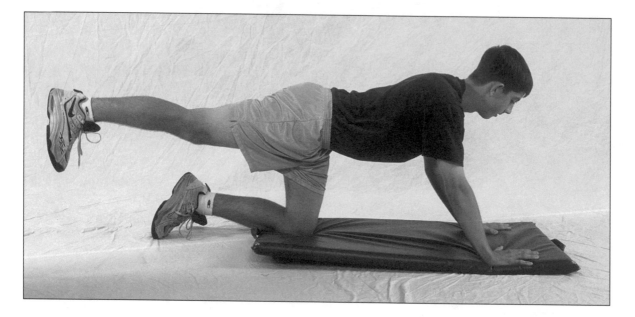

PRONE BACK RAISE

MUSCLES

- Spinal erectors

PROCEDURE

- Lie face down on the floor with a pillow under your hips and abdomen. Extend both arms in front of your head.
- Slowly lift your right leg and left arm until they are a few inches off the floor. Pause momentarily, then return to the starting position. Repeat with your left leg and right arm.

Technique Tips

- Exhale as you lift your limbs upward and inhale as you return your limbs to the starting position.
- Perform this exercise in a slow and controlled manner. Raise your limbs only an inch or two off the floor.

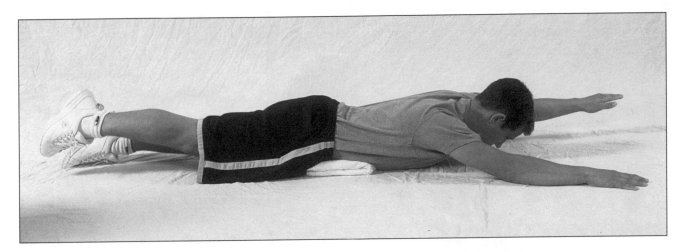

BACK EXTENSION

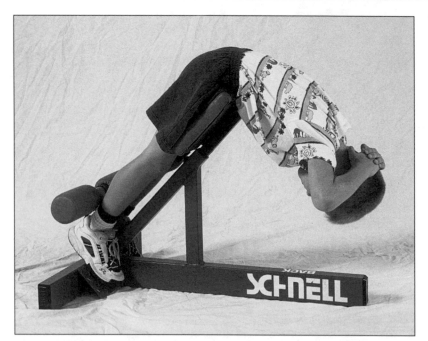

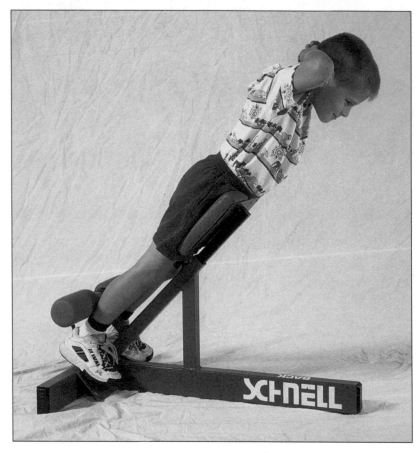

MUSCLES

- Spinal erectors, hip extensors

PROCEDURE

- To position yourself on the equipment, lie in a face down position with your hips resting on the pad and your feet secured under the rear pads. Your navel should be at the far edge of the pad.

- Hang your upper body over the pad, and keep your legs fully extended. It is desirable to round your spine in the lower position. Place your hands behind your head.

- Slowly raise your head and shoulders until your upper body is in line with your lower body; then slowly return to the starting position.

Technique Tips

- Inhale as you lower your body and exhale as you lift it.
- Avoid hyperextending your back at the top of this exercise.
- Be sure that your hips are on the pad.
- To make this exercise easier, place your hands across your chest.
- You may be more comfortable with extra padding (such as a towel) on the edge of the pad.

Summary

Although body-weight training does not require special equipment, some children may not have enough strength to perform selected body-weight exercises. Therefore, we take the time to choose body-weight exercises that are appropriate for each child's strength level because we want children to experience success and feel good about their performance. If necessary, modify a traditional exercise in order to make it easier to perform. Give children an opportunity to learn about body-weight training and gradually add new exercises to their exercise program. Many different body-weight exercises can be used to safely and effectively strengthen all the major muscle groups.

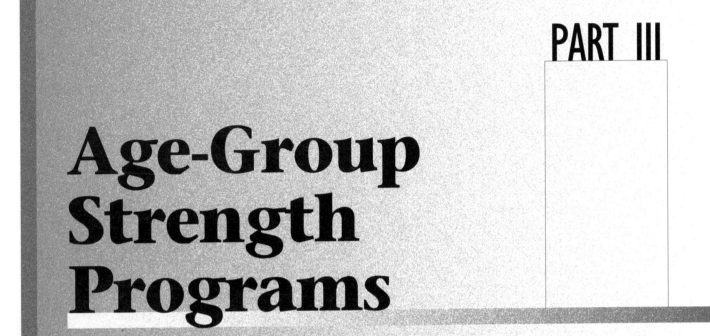

PART III

Age-Group Strength Programs

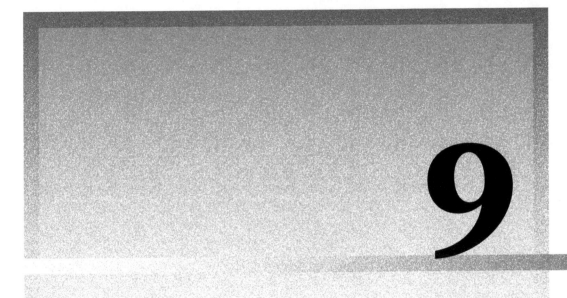

Mighty Mites:
7- to 9-Year-Olds

Our research has shown that boys and girls between 7 and 9 years of age respond positively and enthusiastically to properly designed strength-training programs. Physiologically, our youngest participants have demonstrated significant gains in their muscle strength and exercise performance. Psychologically, they have made impressive improvements in feeling physically competent and self-confident.

We are pleased to report that over the past several years, there have been no injuries or setbacks among our 7- to 9-year-old trainees. Perhaps just as important, the participants in this age group have had an almost zero dropout rate. When the exercise program is interesting and challenging, the children seldom miss a session. Typically, the children's attendance rate is over 95 percent, indicating a high level of personal reinforcement from their strength-training efforts.

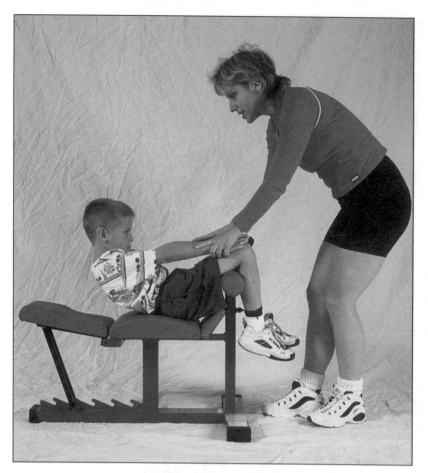

Always take time to emphasize proper technique.

Warm-Up and Cool-Down Components

Be sure to sandwich the strength exercises between warm-up and cool-down segments that feature a variety of physical activities. These include relays, box stepping, rope skipping, active games, agility drills, static and dynamic stretching exercises, and some light strength work with resistance bands. Use balls, hoops, cones, and other apparatus to make these program components more challenging and to enhance the children's locomotor and sport skills.

Strength-Training Program

The youth strength-training guidelines established by the National Strength and Conditioning Association recommend one to three sets of 6 to 15 repetitions, each with appropriate weight loads. Obviously, weight loads that you can perform for only 6 repetitions are much heavier than weight loads for 15 repetitions. Likewise, completing three sets of each exercise is more demanding than doing one set of each exercise. Although it is logical to assume that harder workouts produce better results, 7- to 9-year-old boys and girls respond favorably to brief training sessions and make better strength gains doing higher repetitions (13 to 15) with moderate weight loads.

To effectively condition most major muscle groups, train with 6 to 10 different exercises, two or three days per week. Some of these, such as the leg press and chest press, work several muscles simultaneously, and others, like the hip abduction and hip adduction, target specific muscles. Children in this age group should use a combination of multimuscle and single-muscle exercises that provide comprehensive muscular development. Make sure that children perform every exercise properly, through a full movement range and with slow movement speed.

Machine and Free-Weight Strength-Training Exercises

Table 9.1 presents sample strength exercises for 7- to 9-year-olds using child-sized weight-plate machines, along with a suggested training protocol. If child-sized

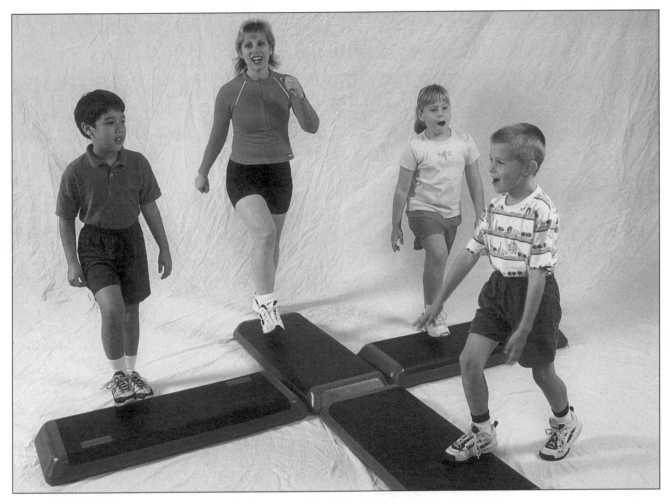

An aerobic warm-up prepares your body for strength-training activities.

resistance machines are not available, you can perform a variety of strength exercises safely and successfully with free-weight equipment. We prefer dumbbells to barbells with this age group for two reasons. First, dumbbell training eliminates the possibility of being trapped under a weighted bar in exercises such as barbell bench presses and barbell squats. Second, dumbbells are easier to hold and handle than barbells, thus enabling children to perform their exercises with more control and confidence. Table 9.2 presents sample strength exercises and training recommendations for 7- to 9-year-olds using dumbbells.

Training Considerations

Some authorities feel strongly that young boys and girls should perform body-weight exercises rather than use external resistance. However, most 7- to 9-year-old children are not strong enough to do standard body-weight exercises, such as push-ups, pull-ups, bar dips, and sit-ups. For this reason, appropriate machine and free-weight exercises in which you can adjust the resistance to each person's strength level are more desirable. For example, an 8-year-old boy may be capable of only 1 push-up but can complete 15 bench presses with eight-pound dumbbells.

TABLE 9.1

Child-Sized Weight Machine Exercises (7-9)

Exercise	Muscle groups	Training sets	Training repetitions	Training frequency
Leg press	Quadriceps Hamstrings Gluteals	1	10-15	2 x week
Leg extension	Quadriceps	1	10-15	2 x week
Leg curl	Hamstrings	1	10-15	2 x week
Chest press	Pectoralis major Front deltoid Triceps	1	10-15	2 x week
Seated row	Latissimus dorsi Rear deltoid Biceps	1	10-15	2 x week
Prone back raise	Erector spinae	1	10-15	2 x week
Trunk curl	Rectus abdominis	1	10-15	2 x week

Although both exercises address the same muscle groups (pectoralis major, front deltoid, triceps), 15 properly performed dumbbell bench presses are obviously safer and more productive than struggling through a single push-up.

Of course, the key to safe and effective strength training is proper exercise form, so youth strength-training instructors must teach and require correct exercise technique at all times. Because some elastic-band exercises are difficult to control, this training equipment may be better suited to older age groups who typically have higher levels of coordination and more experience performing strength exercises than younger participants.

Two things that are essential in working successfully with 7- to 9-year-old boys and girls are competent instruction and careful supervision. Teaching segments must be clear and concise, with brief explanations and perfect demonstrations, so the youth can easily understand and model proper training technique. Even after the children have mastered the exercise performance, observe and interact with them as much as possible throughout each training session to reinforce their exercise efforts and maintain their program enthusiasm. Attention to each participant is the top priority for safe and productive youth strength-training programs.

Please note that you should never permit 7- to 9-year-old boys and girls to lift weights without appropriate supervision. This is especially true for at-home strength exercise, where a comfortable and familiar environment may reduce

TABLE 9.2

Dumbbell Exercises (7-9)				
Exercise	Muscle groups	Training sets	Training repetitions	Training frequency
Dumbbell squat	Quadriceps Hamstrings Gluteals	1	10-15	2 x week
Dumbbell lunge	Quadriceps Hamstrings Gluteals	1	10-15	2 x week
Dumbbell step-up	Quadriceps Hamstrings Gluteals	1	10-15	2 x week
Dumbbell bench press	Pectoralis major Front deltoid Triceps	1	10-15	2 x week
Dumbbell one-arm row	Latissimus dorsi Rear deltoid Biceps	1	10-15	2 x week
Dumbbell lateral raise	Deltoids	1	10-15	2 x week
Prone back raise	Erector spinae	1	*	2 x week
Trunk curl	Rectus abdominis	1	*	2 x week

*Do as many repetitions as you can comfortably complete with body weight.

safety awareness and training seriousness. On the other hand, few physical activities offer as much opportunity for cooperation and mutual assistance as family strength-training sessions. Teaching 7- to 9-year-old youth to do sensible strength exercise is an educational activity that should have long-term health and fitness benefits, especially for those who make strength training a standard component of their personal lifestyle. Age seven is not too young to experience and appreciate the benefits of supervised strength exercise. Just be sure to provide the instruction and attention necessary to ensure safe and successful training sessions. Finally, make every effort to emphasize the fun aspect of exercising with weights.

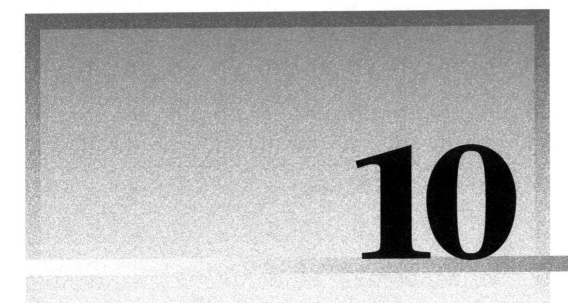

Junior Builders:
10- to 12-Year-Olds

Most of our preadolescent strength-training studies have involved boys and girls in the 10- to 12-year-old range. These are ideal years to start a well-structured and carefully supervised program of resistance exercise. Throughout our 15 years of youth strength-training experience, participants in this age group have consistently demonstrated high levels of interest, ability, and enthusiasm for strength-building exercise. They have also had excellent results, typically increasing their overall muscle strength 50 to 75 percent during the first two months of training. In addition, they have improved their body composition (more muscle and less fat), increased their self-confidence, and enhanced their sport performance.

Warm-Up and Cool-Down Components

Certainly, 10- to 12-year-olds should do other physical activities in addition to strength training. Although some program participants enjoy doing specific endurance exercises, such as stationary cycling or jogging, most boys and girls in this age range prefer a variety of movement activities in a game atmosphere. Therefore, have the children perform many locomotor skills before and after their training session. You may do some warm-up and cool-down activities with music and incorporate apparatus such as balls, hoops, cones, steps, wands, and elastic bands for challenge and variety. Be sure to include several stretching exercises during the warm-up and cool-down segments to enhance joint flexibility. Generally, a one-hour class session should provide about 15 to 20 minutes of warm-up activity, 20 to 25 minutes of strength exercise, and 15 to 20 minutes of cool-down activity.

Strength-Training Program

Although some large 10- to 12-year-olds may fit standard resistance machines, most preteens do better with youth-sized weight machines or dumbbell exercises. The National Strength and Conditioning Association's guidelines of one to three sets of 6 to 15 repetitions are appropriate for this age group, although our participants have had better results training in the 10- to 15-repetition range. Because 10- to 12-year-olds attain similar results with two or three exercise sessions per week, either of these training frequencies will be effective.

Depending on the exercises used, we recommend a program of 6 to 10 different strength exercises. A combination of multiple-muscle exercises, such as bench presses and front pulldowns, and single-muscle exercises, such as biceps curls and triceps pressdowns, may be most effective for addressing all the major muscle groups. Perform all exercises at a controlled movement speed through a full movement range.

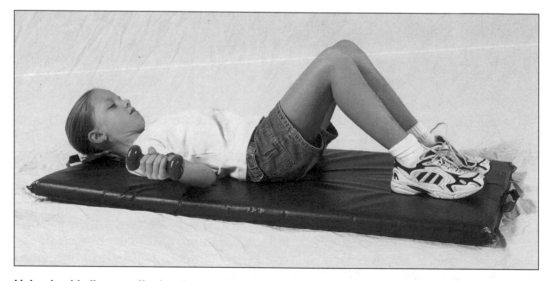

Light dumbbells are effective for a variety of strength exercises.

Machine Strength-Training Exercises

Table 10.1 presents sample strength exercises for 10- to 12-year-old boys and girls using youth-sized weight-stack machines, along with recommendations for training sets, repetitions, and frequency.

TABLE 10.1

Youth-Sized Weight Machine Exercises (10-12)				
Exercise	**Muscle groups**	**Training sets**	**Training repetitions**	**Training frequency**
Leg press	Quadriceps Hamstrings Gluteals	1-2	10-15	2-3 x week
Leg extension	Quadriceps	1	10-15	2-3 x week
Leg curl	Hamstrings	1	10-15	2-3 x week
Chest press	Pectoralis major Front deltoid Triceps	1-2	10-15	2-3 x week
Front pulldown	Latissimus dorsi Rear deltoid Biceps	1-2	10-15	2-3 x week
Overhead press	Deltoids Triceps Upper trapezius	1-2	10-15	2-3 x week
Biceps curl	Biceps	1	10-15	2-3 x week
Triceps pressdown	Triceps	1	10-15	2-3 x week
Hanging-knee raise	Hip flexors Rectus abdominis	1	10-15	2-3 x week
Back extension	Erector spinae	1-2	10-15	2-3 x week
Abdominal curl	Rectus abdominis	1-2	10-15	2-3 x week

Note: If desired, progress to two sets of the multimuscle exercises (leg press, chest press, front pulldown, overhead press) and midsection exercises (back extension, abdominal curl).

Free-Weight Strength-Training Exercises

Although youth-sized resistance machines offer many advantages, 10- to 12-year-old boys and girls can attain excellent results training with free-weight equipment. Because dumbbells are easier to hold and safer to use than barbells, we recommend a basic dumbbell training program for this age group. Table 10.2 presents sample strength exercises and training recommendations for 10- to 12-year-olds using dumbbells.

TABLE 10.2

Dumbbell Exercises (10-12)				
Exercise	Muscle groups	Training sets	Training repetitions	Training frequency
Dumbbell squat	Quadriceps Hamstrings Gluteals	1-2	10-15	2-3 x week
Dumbbell step-up	Quadriceps Hamstrings Gluteals	1-2	10-15	2-3 x week
Dumbbell bench press	Pectoralis major Front deltoid Triceps	1-2	10-15	2-3 x week
Dumbbell one-arm row	Latissimus dorsi Rear deltoid Biceps	1-2	10-15	2-3 x week
Dumbbell incline press	Deltoids Pectoralis major Triceps	1-2	10-15	2-3 x week
Dumbbell incline biceps curl	Biceps	1	10-15	2-3 x week
Dumbbell triceps kickback	Triceps	1	10-15	2-3 x week
Prone back raise	Erector spinae	1-2	*	2-3 x week
Trunk curl	Rectus abdominis	1-2	*	2-3 x week

Note: If desired, progress to two sets of the multimuscle exercises (dumbbell squat, dumbbell step-up, dumbbell bench press, dumbbell one-arm row, dumbbell incline press).

*Do as many repetitions as you can comfortably complete with body weight.

Training Considerations

Some children in the 10- to 12-year-old age group are capable of doing body-weight exercises, such as push-ups and sit-ups. Those who participate in a progressive strength-training program using resistance machines or free weights should find it much easier to perform their body weight exercises. You may include body-weight exercises in the overall conditioning program or use them exclusively if adjustable resistance exercises are not available. Keep in mind that the best way to build muscle strength is by gradually increasing the exercise resistance rather than simply adding more repetitions to fixed-weight movements.

Although push-ups are the standard upper-body exercise, bar dips provide an excellent alternative that addresses the same major muscles (chest, triceps, front shoulders) and places less stress on the lower back. However, heavy boys and girls must be cautious when performing bar dips to make sure they do not descend too far or too fast. Other useful body-weight exercises include trunk curls and hanging-knee raises for the midsection muscles and chin-up modifications for the upper-back and biceps muscles.

The new weight-assisted chin-up and bar dip machines available in most fitness centers enable youth to perform these body-weight exercises with less than body weight. For example, a boy who weighs 70 pounds and places 30 pounds on the weight stack actually lifts 40 pounds of his body weight on each chin-up or bar dip. As he becomes stronger, he may place less weight on the weight stack and use more of his body weight. In this manner, everyone can perform these excellent but challenging exercises and progressively increase the resistance as they develop strength.

Children in this age group may also work with elastic bands, because they typically have sufficient coordination to stabilize their bodies as they perform the exercises. Include a few light resistance band exercises within the warm-up activities.

As with younger boys and girls, the critical factors for safe and successful strength-training experiences are competent instruction and careful

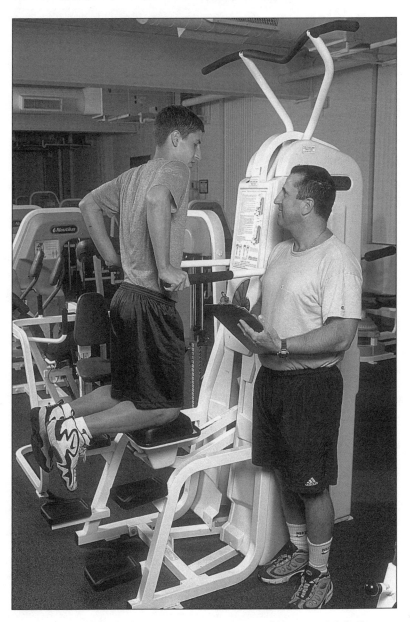

Active supervision is important to prevent accidents and injuries.

supervision. Be sure to introduce each exercise with a concise explanation and precise demonstration. Follow up with careful observation and frequent interaction that include plenty of positive reinforcement for appropriate training behavior.

Although 10- to 12-year-old youth perform well in strength-training classes, do not permit them to exercise in unsupervised settings. In particular, they should do at-home strength training with parents or older brothers and sisters who ensure proper exercise technique and safety awareness.

Most 10- to 12-year-old boys and girls are highly receptive and responsive to structured strength-training programs. Furthermore, children in this age range who do strength exercise are likely to perform other physical activities and make healthy food selections. Every indication is that these are ideal years to introduce young people to the benefits of sensible strength training.

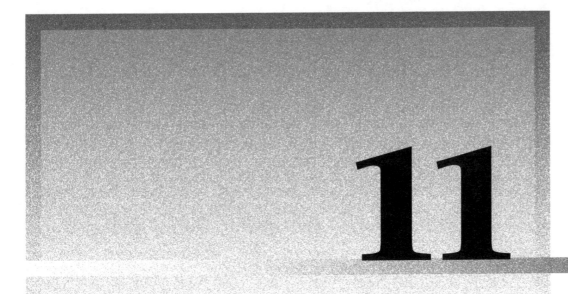

Teens of Steel: 13- to 15-Year-Olds

The early teenage years can be traumatic for boys and girls who experience late physical maturation. This period of transition, commonly called puberty, can be unkind to youth who lag behind their peers in size, strength, or sexual development. Many late bloomers suffer significant loss of self-esteem and feel helpless to change their situations. Although genetics clearly control the growth processes, teens who do strength exercise have certain developmental advantages over those who do not.

Our research with 14-year-olds showed that the boys and girls who strength trained increased their muscle strength by 46 percent compared with only 6 percent for those who did not strength train. Also, during the two-month study period, the training group added four pounds of lean (muscle) weight, while the nontraining group added two pounds of lean (muscle) weight. In addition, the exercisers lost body fat, while the nonexercisers gained body fat. Clearly, the teens who participated in the training program experienced more muscle and strength development than their peers who did not exercise.

Because physical appearance and athletic performance are valued characteristics among most teenagers, sensible strength training can be highly beneficial. On the other hand, teens who aspire to be bodybuilders tend to overtrain by following the high-volume exercise programs presented in popular muscle magazines. These programs typically require dozens of different exercises performed for several sets each. For these reasons, strength-training programs for young teens must be carefully designed to address all major muscle groups with a reasonable number of exercises and moderate workout duration. Adult supervision is essential to encourage the adolescents who are less muscular and underconfident, and to control those who are more muscular and overconfident.

Warm-Up and Cool-Down Components

Generally, teenagers are busy, with plenty of people to see, places to go, and things to do. For these reasons, teen strength-training sessions should be brief, with little wasted time. The warm-up and cool-down components are still important, but you may need to shorten these segments somewhat. Fortunately, teenagers are adept at aerobic activities such as treadmill running, stationary cycling, and stair climbing. To provide both muscular and cardiovascular conditioning in the overall training program, combine about 30 minutes of strength training with about 15 minutes of endurance exercise. Teens are typically willing to perform a few stretching exercises during the warm-up and cool-down periods, and we prefer these components for implementing flexibility exercises.

Strength-Training Program

Most 13- to 15-year-olds are large enough to train on standard resistance machines, especially those that involve pushing or pulling movements such as the leg press, bench press, incline press, overhead press, triceps press, seated row, front pulldown, and weight-assisted chin-up and bar dip machines. They are also capable of executing most free-weight exercises properly and safely, given appropriate instruction and supervision. With careful spotting, young teenagers may perform barbell bench presses and barbell squats, but we definitely prefer the dumbbell versions of these exercises. Both barbell bench presses and barbell squats carry the risk of being pinned beneath a heavy weight load if performed improperly or without a spotter. For this reason, we strongly advise beginning these exercises with an unloaded barbell or even a wooden dowel until the participant develops perfect technique. If you include these lifts in the training program, qualified trainers or training partners must *always* spot them.

Although weight-stack machines offer safety advantages, some teens prefer equipment that uses barbell plates. Plate-loaded equipment is durable and provides a user-friendly combination of free-weight and machine training. Of course, you must take care when loading and unloading the barbell plates. By enforcing the two-hand rule for carrying weight plates, you will greatly reduce the risk of injury from a dropped weight.

The National Strength and Conditioning Association recommends that young teens perform the training exercises for one to three sets of 6 to 15 repetitions each. Table 11.1 presents practical suggestions for designing productive and progressive exercise protocols that are consistent with these strength-training guidelines.

Due to facilities, equipment availability, or philosophy, some teen strength-training programs may emphasize a few (6 to 10) multimuscle free-weight exercises such as the squat, bench press, one-arm row, overhead press, chin-up, or bar dip. As table 11.1 shows, beginners may start with one set of 10 to 15 repetitions and progress to two or three sets of 8 to 12 repetitions after four to eight weeks of training. Generally, we characterize advanced training by more sets, higher weight loads, and fewer repetitions than beginning exercise protocols.

You may also develop teen free-weight training programs around several (11-15) exercises to provide a comparable conditioning effect. In addition to the multimuscle exercises mentioned, such a protocol may include single-muscle exercises such as the biceps curl, triceps extension, lateral raise, trunk curl, or trunk extension. We advise beginners to do one set of 10 to 15 repetitions in

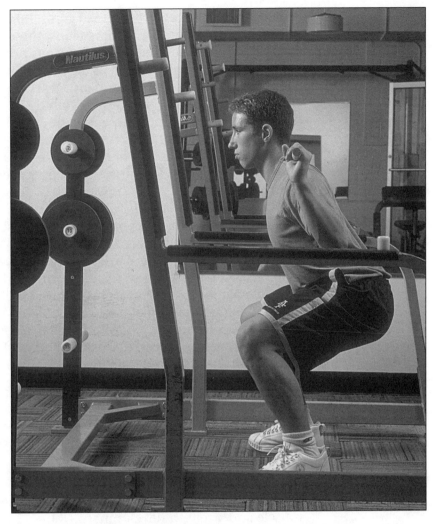

Use a wooden dowel or unloaded barbell when learning and practicing free-weight exercises such as the squat.

TABLE 11.1

Guidelines for Designing Strength-Training Protocols for 13- to 15-Year-Olds Using Various Types of Exercise Equipment				
Exercise equipment	Sets	Beginning repetitions	Sets	Advanced repetitions
Free weights 6-10 exercises	1	10-15	2-3	8-12
Free weights 11-15 exercises	1	10-15	1-2	8-12
Machines 6-10 exercises	1	10-15	2-3	8-12
Machines 11-15 exercises	1	10-15	1-2	8-12

each exercise (see table 11.1). As training progresses, two sets of 8 to 12 repetitions may be advisable. For some teens, three sets of each exercise may be appropriate as long as the total training time is not excessive.

Like the free-weight protocols, teens who work with machines may emphasize a few multimuscle exercises or perform several single muscle exercises to ensure a well-rounded training program. As table 11.1 indicates, teens doing 6 to 10 machine exercises should begin with one set of 10 to 15 repetitions each. As their muscular conditioning improves, they may add a second or third set, and increase the exercise resistance to the 8- to 12-repetition range. The standard multimuscle machines include the leg press, bench press, seated row, incline press, pulldown, overhead press, or weight-assisted chin up and bar dip.

Teens who follow an 11- to 15-machine training program should attain excellent results by performing one or two good sets of each exercise, although they may complete three if desired (see table 11.1). We recommend doing 10 to 15 repetitions during the first few weeks of training, then raising the resistance so participants can complete 8 to 12 repetitions with proper technique. Typical single-muscle machine exercises for this training protocol include the leg extension, leg curl, hip adduction, hip abduction, pullover, lateral raise, biceps curl, triceps extension, back extension, abdominal curl, or rotary torso. Teens involved in sports should also perform neck extensions and neck flexions to condition this vulnerable area of the body and thereby reduce the risk of catastrophic injury. Of course, there is nothing wrong with a workout program that combines several single-muscle and multiple-muscle exercises.

Machine and Free-Weight Strength-Training Exercises

Although many combinations of productive free-weight and machine training protocols are possible, tables 11.2-11.5 represent good starting points for overall muscle and strength development. Table 11.2 presents 8 basic free-weight exercises for 13- to 15-year-olds that address most major muscle groups. If facilities and equipment permit more free-weight exercises, start with the 12-exercise training protocol presented in table 11.3. Young teens who train with machines should attain good results with the basic eight-station program presented in table 11.4. If a variety of resistance machines are available, you can achieve a comprehensive muscle-conditioning program with the 14-station protocol presented in table 11.5.

Training Considerations

Encourage young teens to handle their body weight in challenging exercises such as chin-ups and bar dips. If weight-assisted chin-up and bar-dip equipment is available, start on these machines to encourage the exercise experience. For example, a 14-year-old girl who cannot lift her full body weight of 100 pounds may start with 60 pounds by placing 40 pounds on the weight stack. As she becomes stronger, she can train with 70 pounds of her body weight by placing 30 pounds on the weight stack. In other words, by systematically placing less weight on the weight stack, she can progressively increase her strength until she is lifting her full body weight.

TABLE 11.2

Free Weight Exercises—8 Stations (13-15)				
Exercise	Muscle groups	Training sets	Training repetitions	Training frequency
Barbell squat	Quadriceps Hamstrings Gluteals	2-3	8-12	2-3 x week
Barbell bench press	Pectoralis major Front deltoid Triceps	2-3	8-12	2-3 x week
Dumbbell one-arm row	Latissimus dorsi Rear deltoid Biceps	2-3	8-12	2-3 x week
Dumbbell overhead press	Deltoids Triceps	2-3	8-12	2-3 x week
Chin-up	Latissimus dorsi Rear deltoid Biceps	2-3	*	2-3 x week
Bar dip	Pectoralis major Front deltoid Triceps	2-3	*	2-3 x week
Prone back raise	Erector spinae	2-3	*	2-3 x week
Trunk curl	Rectus abdominis	2-3	*	2-3 x week

Note: Remember to begin with one set of 10 to 15 repetitions before progressing to two or three sets of 8 to 12 repetitions.

*Do as many repetitions as you can comfortably complete with body weight.

The ability to handle their body weight in chin-ups and bar dips typically increases a teen's self-confidence and provides positive reinforcement to their training efforts from a practical perspective.

Thirteen- to 15-year-old youth can certainly train with elastic bands safely and effectively. This type of training may be useful in class settings or on the field for sport teams as it is light, portable, and easy to use. Elastic bands are inexpensive, but it is important to have bands of varying resistance for each trainee to accommodate muscle abilities in different exercises. For example, heavier bands for leg exercises and lighter bands for arm exercises.

Although it is tempting to assume that athletic teens can attain high levels of muscular fitness through sport participation, this is seldom the case. In fact, to

TABLE 11.3

Free Weight Exercises—12 Stations (13-15)

Exercise	Muscle groups	Training sets	Training repetitions	Training frequency
Barbell squat	Quadriceps Hamstrings Gluteals	1-2	8-12	2-3 x week
Dumbbell step-up	Quadriceps Hamstrings Gluteals	1-2	8-12	2-3 x week
Barbell bench press	Pectoralis major Front deltoid Triceps	1-2	8-12	2-3 x week
Dumbbell one-arm row	Latissimus dorsi Rear deltoid Biceps	1-2	8-12	2-3 x week
Dumbbell overhead press	Deltoids Triceps	1-2	8-12	2-3 x week
Dumbbell biceps curl	Biceps	1-2	8-12	2-3 x. week
Dumbbell triceps overhead extension	Triceps	1-2	8-12	2-3 x week
Dumbbell shrug	Upper trapezius	1-2	8-12	2-3 x week
Bar dip	Pectoralis major Front deltoid Triceps	1-2	*	2-3 x week
Chin-up	Latissimus dorsi Rear deltoid Biceps	1-2	*	2-3 x week
Prone back raise	Erector spinae	1-2	*	2-3 x week
Trunk curl	Rectus abdominis	1-2	*	2-3 x week

Note: Remember to begin with one set of 10 to 15 repetitions before progressing to two sets of 8 to 12 repetitions.

*Do as many repetitions as you can comfortably complete with body weight.

TABLE 11.4

Resistance Machine Exercises—8 Stations (13-15)				
Exercise	Muscle groups	Training sets	Training repetitions	Training frequency
Leg press	Quadriceps Hamstrings Gluteals	2-3	8-12	2-3 x week
Chest press	Pectoralis major Front deltoid Triceps	2-3	8-12	2-3 x week
Seated row	Latissimus dorsi Rear deltoid Biceps	2-3	8-12	2-3 x week
Overhead press	Deltoids Triceps	2-3	8-12	2-3 x week
Weight-assisted chin-up	Latissimus dorsi Rear deltoid Biceps	2-3	8-12	2-3 x week
Weight-assisted bar dip	Pectoralis major Front deltoid Triceps	2-3	8-12	2-3 x week
Low-back extension	Erector spinae	2-3	8-12	2-3 x week
Rotary torso	Obliques Rectus abdominis	2-3	8-12	2-3 x week

Note: Remember to begin with one set of 10 to 15 repetitions before progressing to two sets of 8 to 12 repetitions.

minimize injury risk and maximize performance potential, young athletes should participate in well-designed strength-training programs that provide comprehensive muscle conditioning. The training protocols presented in this chapter address all major muscle groups in a balanced manner and are most appropriate for young athletes.

After receiving proper exercise instruction and demonstrating desirable training technique, most teens can function independently in supervised fitness centers. Even under supervised conditions, however, it may be necessary to remind teens of safe and sensible strength-training procedures. Young teens should not compete with each other, use maximum weight loads, or compromise their exercise form under any circumstances.

TABLE 11.5

Resistance Machine Exercises—14 Stations (13-15)

Exercise	Muscle groups	Training sets	Training repetitions	Training frequency
Leg press	Quadriceps Hamstrings Gluteals	1-2	8-12	2-3 x week
Leg extension	Quadriceps	1-2	8-12	2-3 x week
Leg curl	Hamstrings	1-2	8-12	2-3 x week
Hip adduction	Hip adductors	1-2	8-12	2-3 x week
Hip abduction	Hip abductors	1-2	8-12	2-3 x week
Chest press	Pectoralis major Front deltoid Triceps	1-2	8-12	2-3 x week
Seated row	Latissimus dorsi Rear deltoid Biceps	1-2	8-12	2-3 x week
Overhead press	Deltoids Triceps	1-2	8-12	2-3 x week
Biceps curl	Biceps	1-2	8-12	2-3 x week
Triceps extension	Triceps	1-2	8-12	2-3 x week
Weight-assisted chin-up	Latissimus dorsi Rear deltoid Biceps	1-2	8-12	2-3 x week
Weight-assisted bar dip	Pectoralis major Front deltoid Triceps	1-2	8-12	2-3 x week
Low-back extension	Erector spinae	1-2	8-12	2-3 x week
Abdominal curl	Rectus abdominis	1-2	8-12	2-3 x week

Note: Begin with one set of 10 to 15 repetitions before progressing to two sets of 8 to 12 repetitions.

PART IV

Strength Programs for Sports

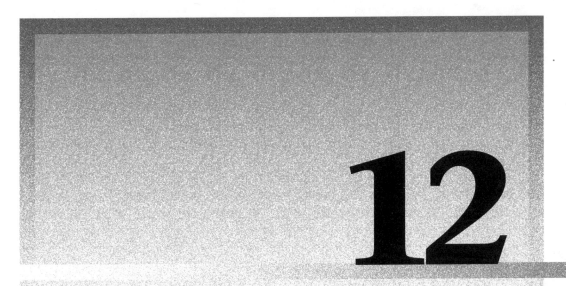

General Sport-Conditioning Programs

The key to successful sport conditioning is a well-designed strength-training program that promotes balanced development of the major muscle groups. Although different sports have different conditioning requirements, young athletes should complete a general muscle-conditioning program before beginning sport-specific strength training. By first developing high strength levels in all major muscle groups, athletes greatly reduce the risk of injuries. On the other hand, if individuals address only the muscles used most in a particular sport or athletic event, these muscles are more likely to experience overuse injuries, and the untrained muscles are more prone to traumatic injuries.

Perhaps the following examples will illustrate the importance of overall muscle conditioning for safe and productive sport experiences. One of the authors has coached track and cross country at the junior high, high school, and college levels. One year, he determined that his sprinters should train specifically to explode out of the starting blocks and to avoid injured (pulled) hamstring muscles. He had them do several strength-training exercises for their quadriceps (front thigh) muscles, which are responsible for fast starts. He also had them perform lots of stretching exercises for their hamstrings (rear thigh) muscles, which are typically susceptible to pulls but he did strength train for these muscles. Although this approach seemed to make sense from an event-specific approach, it produced disastrous results. As the track season progressed, all the sprinters experienced pulled hamstrings muscles. The underlying problem was a muscle imbalance created by strengthening the quadriceps muscles without also strengthening the opposing hamstring muscles. Because the weaker hamstring muscles could not effectively counteract the stronger quadriceps muscles during the explosive sprinting action, they were overpowered and injured (pulled).

The knowledge gained from this unfortunate training experience was helpful in designing a balanced program of strength exercise for a girls' cross country and track team. The teens on this team did one exercise for each major muscle group to achieve a comprehensive or total-body conditioning effect. Table 12.1 presents the training exercises and target muscle groups this strength program addressed.

The athletes performed one set of each exercise, requiring about 30 minutes to complete the workout. They trained three days a week throughout the off-season months (winter and summer). This overall approach to muscle conditioning was highly successful. Over a four-year period, the 30 girls on coach George Rose's team encountered only one injury and won four consecutive New England cross country championships. Clearly, this basic and balanced strength-training program played a large role in preventing running injuries and at least a small role in improving the athletes' running performance.

Based on this and numerous other programs with youth sport participants, a comprehensive muscle-conditioning program is essential for successful athletic experiences, and athletes should complete it before sport-specific strength training. That is, young athletes should complete the overall power and strength-building programs presented in this chapter (medicine ball exercises plus free weights or machines) before jumping into sport-specific training programs featured in the following chapters (see tables 12.2 through 12.7, pages 166-171). We recommend one month each of the beginning, intermediate, and advanced programs before sport-specific training. Remember to build a broad base of muscle strength before initiating sport-specific exercise protocols.

Power Training for General Sport Conditioning

Successful sport performance requires a combination of strength and power. Although most conditioning programs for young athletes highlight the importance of specific strength-building exercises, don't overlook the value of power training. Although strength training can make muscles stronger, power training can develop explosiveness or speed. Medicine ball exercises are ideal for power training because you can perform the exercises quickly.

TABLE 12.1

Notre Dame High School Cross Country Team Strength-Training Exercises

Strength-training exercises	Target muscle groups
Leg extension	Quadriceps (front thigh)
Leg curl	Hamstrings (rear thigh)
Hip adduction	Hip adductors (inner thigh)
Hip abduction	Hip abductors (outer thigh)
Chest press	Pectoralis major (chest)
Pullover	Latissimus dorsi (upper back)
Lateral raise	Deltoids (shoulders)
Biceps curl	Biceps (front arm)
Triceps extension	Triceps (rear arm)
Abdominal curl	Rectus abdominis (midsection)
Low-back extension	Erector spinae (lower back)
Neck flexion	Neck flexors (front neck)
Neck extension	Neck extensors (rear neck)

Further, you can use a variety of medicine ball exercises consisting of throwing and jumping movements to condition the total body in a short time. If you have never used medicine balls before, master the technique of each exercise before you attempt to perform these exercises explosively. Of course, be sure to warm up by performing several minutes of aerobic exercise and stretching before power training. Incorporate lightweight medicine ball exercises into the warm-up period, and always allow the participants to perform a few practice repetitions of an exercise before the power-training session begins. With appropriate instruction and a training partner, young athletes will find these exercises challenging and fun. Remember, to generate near-maximal power during the workout, perform the power exercises before the strength exercises.

Strength Training for General Sport Conditioning

The following information should help you design safe and effective sport-conditioning programs using free-weight or machine exercises.

Legs

Most sports involve running and jumping, so a major emphasis of the conditioning program should be strengthening exercises for the large, propulsive muscles of the thigh. These include the quadriceps, hamstrings, and gluteals. Free-weight training is effective for working these muscle groups together by using squats, step-ups, and lunges. Squats are the safest of these exercises due to the fixed feet position and stable base of support.

Machine training can also address the three major leg muscle groups (quadriceps, hamstrings, gluteals) simultaneously by using the leg press exercise. You can also train the thigh muscles individually through the leg extension (quadriceps) and leg curl exercises (hamstrings). In addition, you can effectively train the leg muscles responsible for lateral movements on machines. You can work the inner-thigh muscles on the hip adduction machine and the outer-thigh muscles on the hip abduction machine.

Trunk

Sports that involve throwing or striking movements require efficient transfer of forces from the power muscles of the legs to the performance muscles of the upper body. The major muscles responsible for this force transfer are the erector spinae muscles of the lower back, the rectus abdominis muscles in the front midsection, and the oblique muscles on both sides of the midsection.

You can strengthen these muscles by body-weight exercises, such as the prone back raise for the lower back and diagonal trunk curls for the midsection groups. You can also train them on the following resistance machines: low-back extension, abdominal curl, and rotary torso.

Upper Body

Although the upper body consists of many muscles, the most important areas are the chest (pectoralis major), upper back (latissimus dorsi), and shoulders (deltoids). Traditional free-weight exercises for these muscles are the barbell bench press, dumbbell one-arm row, and dumbbell overhead press. Typical machine exercises include the chest press, seated row, and overhead press.

Upper Arms

You can exercise the upper-arm muscles effectively with free weights and machines. The standard exercises with both modes of training are biceps curls for the biceps muscles and triceps extensions for the triceps muscles.

Neck

Because the neck is vulnerable to injury, we strongly recommend that young athletes train the neck flexor and extensor muscles. With free-weights, you can use the dumbbell shrug exercise to work the upper trapezius muscle that runs from the head to the upper back and shoulders. The four-way neck machine provides a most effective means for safely strengthening the muscles in the back, front, and sides of the neck.

Exercise Programs for General Sport Conditioning

This section presents two progressive strength- and power-training programs for conditioning young athletes. Perform program one with free weights, doing one month of basic training, one month of intermediate training, and one month of advanced training (see tables 12.2 through 12.4). Program two follows the same training format, but you perform it with resistance machines (see tables 12.5 through 12.7). Both programs should begin with power-training exercises. For basic training, perform one set of 6 to 10 repetitions on the medicine ball chest pass and underhand throw exercises.

Try a lightweight medicine ball at first (about two pounds for children and four pounds for teenagers), and work on developing the technique of each exercise. Unlike strength-building exercises, you should perform power exercises quickly. Focus on increasing the speed of each exercise and the distance you throw the ball. As you progress to intermediate and advanced levels of training, perform two, then three sets of these exercises. Remember, because movement speed is fundamental to developing power, don't sacrifice speed for a heavy ball. When performing more than one set on a strength or power exercise, the young athlete should rest one to two minutes between sets.

Applying the
Strength- and Power-Training Programs

The suggested strength- and power-training programs presented in this chapter serve only as samples that you may adjust according to the athlete's age and training objectives, as well as for available facilities and equipment. The progression from beginning, to intermediate, to advanced programs may be longer or shorter than the recommended one-month training phases. In fact, it is acceptable to stay with the time-efficient beginner program throughout the entire conditioning period. Simply increasing the exercise resistance by about five percent whenever the athlete completes 15 repetitions provides a productive stimulus for progressive muscle and strength development.

The key to successful sport conditioning is knowing when to change the training protocol. Generally, young athletes should continue their training program until progress begins to plateau. They should then switch to a different exercise protocol that provides a new stimulus for further muscle and strength gains. In addition to the medicine ball exercises described in this book, you can use your imagination to create new medicine ball exercises that meet your sport-specific needs.

Although the basic strength- and power-training programs presented in this chapter provide comprehensive muscle conditioning that applies to all athletic activities, various sports may benefit from specialized strength exercises. To this end, the following chapters present sport-specific training protocols that may supplement the general strength- and power-conditioning programs. We group these training protocols according to the major emphasis of the sports, namely, power, endurance, jumping, or striking. Be sure the young athletic participants

TABLE 12.2

General Conditioning Using Free Weights—Beginners

Exercise	Muscle groups	Training sets	Training repetitions	Training frequency
Barbell squat	Quadriceps Hamstrings Gluteals	1	10-15	2 x week
Barbell bench press	Pectoralis major Front deltoid Triceps	1	10-15	2 x week
Dumbbell one-arm row	Latissimus dorsi Rear deltoid Biceps	1	10-15	2 x week
Dumbbell overhead press	Deltoids Triceps	1	10-15	2 x week
Dumbbell biceps curl	Biceps	1	10-15	2 x week
Dumbbell triceps overhead extension	Triceps	1	10-15	2 x week
Trunk curl	Rectus abdominis	1	*	2 x week
Prone back raise	Erector spinae	1	*	2 x week

*Do as many repetitions as you can comfortably complete with body weight.

TABLE 12.3

General Conditioning Using Free Weights—Intermediate

Exercise	Muscle groups	Training sets	Training repetitions	Training frequency
Barbell squat	Quadriceps Hamstrings Gluteals	1-2	8-12	2-3 x week
Dumbbell step-up	Quadriceps Hamstrings Gluteals	1-2	8-12	2-3 x week
Barbell bench press	Pectoralis major Front deltoid Triceps	1-2	8-12	2-3 x week
Dumbbell one-arm row	Latissimus dorsi Rear deltoid Biceps	1-2	8-12	2-3 x week
Dumbbell incline press	Deltoids Upper pectoralis major Triceps	1-2	8-12	2-3 x week
Dumbbell incline biceps curl	Biceps	1-2	8-12	2-3 x week
Dumbbell triceps overhead extension	Triceps	1-2	8-12	2-3 x week
Dumbbell shrug	Upper trapezius	1-2	8-12	2-3 x week
Trunk curl	Rectus abdominis	1-2	*	2-3 x week
Prone back raise	Erector spinae	1-2	*	2-3 x week

*Do as many repetitions as you can comfortably complete with body weight.

TABLE 12.4

General Conditioning Using Free Weights—Advanced

Exercise	Muscle groups	Training sets	Training repetitions	Training frequency
Barbell squat	Quadriceps Hamstrings Gluteals	2-3	6-10	2-3 x week
Dumbbell step-up	Quadriceps Hamstrings Gluteals	2-3	6-10	2-3 x week
Barbell bench press	Pectoralis major Front deltoid Triceps	2-3	6-10	2-3 x week
Dumbbell one-arm row	Latissimus dorsi Rear deltoid Biceps	2-3	6-10	2-3 x week
Dumbbell incline press	Deltoids Upper pectoralis major Triceps	2-3	6-10	2-3 x week
Dumbbell incline biceps curl	Biceps	2-3	6-10	2-3 x week
Dumbbell triceps overhead extension	Triceps	2-3	6-10	2-3 x week
Dumbbell shrug	Upper trapezius	2-3	6-10	2-3 x week
Bar dip	Pectoralis major Front deltoid Triceps	2-3	*	2-3 x week
Chin-up	Latissimus dorsi Rear deltoid Biceps	2-3	*	2-3 x week
Prone back raise	Erector spinae	2-3	*	2-3 x week
Trunk curl	Rectus abdominis	2-3	*	2-3 x week

Note: If the training facility has a pulley apparatus, substitute pulldowns for dumbbell one-arm rows and pressdowns for dumbbell triceps overhead extensions.

*Do as many repetitions as you can comfortably complete with body weight.

TABLE 12.5

General Conditioning Using Resistance Machines—Beginners

Exercise	Muscle groups	Training sets	Training repetitions	Training frequency
Leg press	Quadriceps Hamstrings Gluteals	1	10-15	2 x week
Chest press	Pectoralis major Front deltoid Triceps	1	10-15	2 x week
Seated row	Latissimus dorsi Rear deltoid Biceps	1	10-15	2 x week
Overhead press	Deltoids Triceps	1	10-15	2 x week
Weight-assisted chin-up	Latissimus dorsi Rear deltoid Biceps	1	10-15	2 x week
Weight-assisted bar dip	Pectoralis major Front deltoid Triceps	1	10-15	2 x week
Low-back extension	Erector spinae	1	10-15	2 x week
Abdominal curl	Rectus abdominis	1	10-15	2 x week

TABLE 12.6

General Conditioning Using Resistance Machines—Intermediate

Exercise	Muscle groups	Training sets	Training repetitions	Training frequency
Leg press	Quadriceps Hamstrings Gluteals	1-2	8-12	2-3 x week
Leg extension	Quadriceps	1-2	8-12	2-3 x week
Leg curl	Hamstrings	1-2	8-12	2-3 x week
Chest press	Pectoralis major Front deltoid Triceps	1-2	8-12	2-3 x week
Seated row	Latissimus dorsi Rear deltoid Biceps	1-2	8-12	2-3 x week
Overhead press	Deltoids Triceps	1-2	8-12	2-3 x week
Weight-assisted chin-up	Latissimus dorsi Rear deltoid Biceps	1-2	8-12	2-3 x week
Weight-assisted bar dip	Pectoralis major Front deltoid Triceps	1-2	8-12	2-3 x week
Low-back extension	Erector spinae	1-2	8-12	2-3 x week
Abdominal curl	Rectus abdominis	1-2	8-12	2-3 x week
Neck extension	Neck extensors	1-2	8-12	2-3 x week
Neck flexion	Neck flexors	1-2	8-12	2-3 x week

TABLE 12.7

General Conditioning Using Resistance Machines—Advanced

Exercise	Muscle groups	Training sets	Training repetitions	Training frequency
Leg press	Quadriceps Hamstrings Gluteals	2-3	6-10	2-3 x week
Leg extension	Quadriceps	2-3	6-10	2-3 x week
Leg curl	Hamstrings	2-3	6-10	2-3 x week
Hip adduction	Hip adductors	2-3	6-10	2-3 x week
Hip abduction	Hip abductors	2-3	6-10	2-3 x week
Chest press	Pectoralis major Front deltoid Triceps	2-3	6-10	2-3 x week
Seated row	Latissimus dorsi Rear deltoid Biceps	2-3	6-10	2-3 x week
Overhead press	Deltoids Triceps	2-3	6-10	2-3 x week
Biceps curl	Biceps	2-3	6-10	2-3 x week
Triceps extension	Triceps	2-3	6-10	2-3 x week
Weight-assisted chin-up	Latissimus dorsi Rear deltoid Biceps	2-3	6-10	2-3 x week
Weight-assisted bar dip	Pectoralis major Front deltoid Triceps	2-3	6-10	2-3 x week
Low-back extension	Erector spinae	2-3	6-10	2-3 x week
Abdominal curl	Rectus abdominis	2-3	6-10	2-3 x week
Neck extension	Neck extensors	2-3	6-10	2-3 x week
Neck flexion	Neck flexors	2-3	6-10	2-3 x week

GENERAL SPORTS

continue their basic strength-training program, and use the sport-specific exercises as additions rather than substitutions.

As you use the sport-specific training protocols in appendix A (free weights) and appendix B (weight machines), please note that the exercises are listed in order from larger to smaller muscle groups. Exercises for the legs are presented first, followed by exercises for the chest, upper back, shoulders, arms, lower back, abdominals, neck, shoulder rotator cuff, and forearms. Medicine ball exercises that address many major muscle groups together are presented last. You should find the exercise tables easy to understand and implement.

13

Power Sports: Football, Rugby, Wrestling, Gymnastics, Track and Field

Participants in power activities such as football, rugby, wrestling, gymnastics, track and field should be well-prepared for successful sport performance by following the general strength and conditioning programs in chapter 12. These programs address the major muscle groups in a balanced manner to increase overall strength and reduce injury risk.

However, power sports have certain requirements that you may better achieve by adding specific power and strength exercises. Most of these sports use muscles of the legs, chest, and arms in a pronounced pushing action. Although squats, bench presses and incline presses are highly effective for conditioning these muscles, it is unwise to perform these exercises explosively. For power development, use medicine ball drills in which you can accelerate and release the ball in a forceful pushing movement. Medicine ball underhand throws, squat tosses, and chest passes seem well suited for improving power production in the pushing muscles. The following sections present supplementary strength-building exercises and sample training protocols for various sports characterized by power production.

Football and Rugby

Because football and rugby have so many similarities, especially with respect to muscular power, we grouped these activities together. Sprinting and blocking depend on leg power, which you can enhance by performing lunges, heel raises, barbell squats, and leg presses.

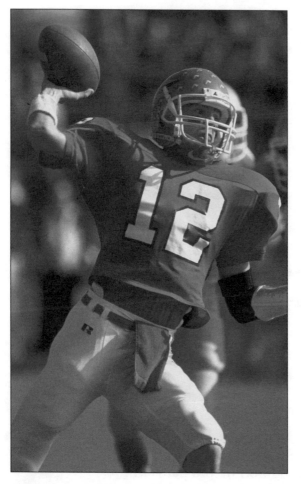

Football players need strength and power to be successful.

Lunges, like squats and step-ups, involve the quadriceps, hamstrings, and gluteal muscles. However, they have a ballistic action, with pronounced deceleration (stepping forward) and acceleration (pushing backward) phases. Although you can effectively perform lunges with barbells and dumbbells, the latter is more appropriate for young athletes. It is certainly safer to do lunges while holding dumbbells than with a barbell across the back.

Heel raises address the gastrocnemius and soleus muscles of the calves, and you can perform them with dumbbells, barbells, or machines. However, they have greater impact on the large gastrocnemius muscle when you do them from a straight-leg rather than a bent-knee position.

Hip extension depends on the hamstring and gluteal muscles, and you can address this with progressive resistance in exercises such as barbell squats and leg presses.

Due to the potential for catastrophic injury to the neck, it is essential to condition the neck muscles of young football and rugby players. The first choice for safe and progressive strengthening of the neck muscles is the four-way neck machine. This resistance apparatus addresses the extensor (rear), flexor (front), and lateral flexor (side) muscles of the neck. If the four-way neck machine is not available, the dumbbell shrug exercise effectively works the upper trapezius muscle in the rear neck and upper-back area.

Strong forearm muscles are important for tackling, gripping the football, and reducing the risk of wrist injuries. The super-forearm machine provides five separate exercises for the flexor, extensor, pronator, supinator, and finger-gripping muscles of the forearms. If this training tool is unavailable, you can achieve excellent forearm conditioning by performing the wrist roller exercise with a homemade pipe, rope, and weight-plate apparatus (see chapter 5 for exercise description and illustration).

Wrestling

If there are any sports that use all muscles of the body, then wrestling is certainly at the top of the list. Wrestlers should perform a variety of exercises for comprehensive muscular conditioning. However, the rigors of this sport call for special attention to the neck and midsection muscles, as well as the gripping muscles of the forearms, and the lunging muscles of the legs. If available, use the four-way neck machine to strengthen the muscles in the front, back, and sides of the neck. The preferred free-weight exercise is the dumbbell shrug which targets the upper trapezius muscles involved in neck extension.

In addition to strong low-back and abdominal muscles, wrestlers require fully functional oblique muscles for turning themselves and their opponents. The rotary torso machine is ideal for working the internal and external obliques on both sides of the midsection. In the absence of this machine, diagonal trunk curls performed on the floor or an incline board can effectively condition the oblique muscles.

Because a viselike grip is most valuable in controlling an opponent, wrestlers should spend some extra time working their forearm muscles. The super-forearm machine addresses all the muscles involved in gripping and wrist movements. The recommended free-weight alternative is the wrist roller exercise that requires a pipe, a short section of rope, and a 5- or 10-pound barbell plate (see chapter 5 for exercise description and illustration).

The lunging action involved in many takedowns makes dumbbell lunges relevant for wrestlers. We recommend this exercise for event-specific strengthening of the quadriceps, hamstrings, and gluteal muscles.

Gymnastics

Although some events are different, there is much similarity between boys' and girls' gymnastics, and athletes can use the same strength-training program for conditioning. Leg power is essential for floor exercise, vaulting, and balance beam. We recommend the leg press, squat, and dumbbell lunge for conditioning the hip and thigh muscles, and the heel raise (machine or barbell) works well for strengthening the calf muscles.

Grip strength is critical for the high bar, side horse, parallel bars, and uneven bars. The super-forearm machine is best suited for overall forearm conditioning, which results in greater grip strength. If this apparatus is unavailable, use wrist curls and wrist extensions performed with dumbbells.

All gymnastics events require strong midsection muscles, including the obliques and hip flexors. You can effectively exercise the oblique muscles with the rotary torso machine or diagonal trunk curls. You can condition the hip flexor muscles by performing hanging-knee raises on dip bars.

POWER SPORTS

Track and Field

Many track and field events are power activities that may benefit from specialized training. Sprinters, jumpers, and throwers all need powerful leg muscles. Consider adding the dumbbell lunge exercise for greater hip and thigh strength, and the heel raise (machine or barbell) for conditioning the calf muscles.

Throwers and pole-vaulters require high levels of upper-body strength, especially in the pushing muscles of the chest, shoulders, and triceps. Both the machine chest press and the dumbbell incline press serve this purpose well. These athletes will certainly benefit from powerful chest passes with medicine balls of varying weights.

Throwers and pole-vaulters also need strong midsection muscles to effectively transfer forces from the legs to the upper body. The rotary torso machine and diagonal trunk curl address the muscles in the front and sides of the midsection and should facilitate leg to upper-body force transfer.

These same athletes must have good grip strength to securely grasp the shot, discus, javelin, or vaulting pole. The super-forearm machine works all muscles involved in wrist movements and gripping. If this machine is not accessible, wrist curls and wrist extensions performed with dumbbells provide similar training effects.

Pole-vaulters and jumpers initiate their upward movement with a powerful hip flexion action. They should therefore perform hanging-knee raises from dip bars.

Applying Power Sports Exercise Programs

Please keep in mind that the suggested sport-specific exercise programs are not rigid guidelines, and you may alter them for different athletes and training circumstances. Feel free to add, subtract, or substitute exercises as necessary due to time constraints, equipment availability, and conditioning objectives.

Generally, power- and strength-training protocols should be effective with one to three sets per exercise. On the machine and free-weight exercises, repetition ranges should progress from higher to lower as muscle strength increases. Begin with 10 to 15 repetitions per set; then use more resistance for 8 to 12 repetitions per set. On the power exercises, perform 6 to 10 repetitions per set, and increase the speed of the exercise movements before you increase the weight of the medicine ball (see appendixes A and B for sport-specific exercises).

We designed the conditioning program to enhance power production by performing the strength exercises with controlled movement speed through a full movement range. The only exercises that you should execute quickly are the medicine ball drills, as you can accelerate these movements through the point of ball release.

Although young sport participants may train three days per week during the off-season, they should cut back to two workouts per week during the competitive period. The rigors of sport activity may make it difficult to achieve full muscle recovery when doing demanding strength exercises every other day. Our research clearly shows that two training sessions per week produce almost as much strength gain and muscle development as three weekly workouts.

Sport coaches should be present and actively involved in each strength-training session. It is important to encourage good training effort, to ensure correct exercise technique, and to reinforce appropriate weight-room attitudes and actions.

Jumping Sports: Basketball, Volleyball, Netball, Dance, Figure Skating

The general strength and conditioning programs presented in chapter 12 should establish an excellent base from which to enhance jumping ability in sports such as basketball, volleyball, netball, dance, and figure skating. The overall training approach provides comprehensive muscle conditioning and balanced strength development to increase performance potential and decrease injury risk.

Nonetheless, sports that require plenty of powerful jumps may benefit from specialized training and specific power and strength exercises. For power development in the lower extremities, use medicine ball drills such as squat tosses, underhand throws, and lunge passes. These exercises condition the legs to perform quickly and explosively. The sections that follow offer training programs and supplementary exercises to strengthen the jumping muscles. Proper performance of the power and strength workouts should improve both jumping quality and quantity. That is, young athletes should be able to jump higher and perform successive jumps with less loss of power.

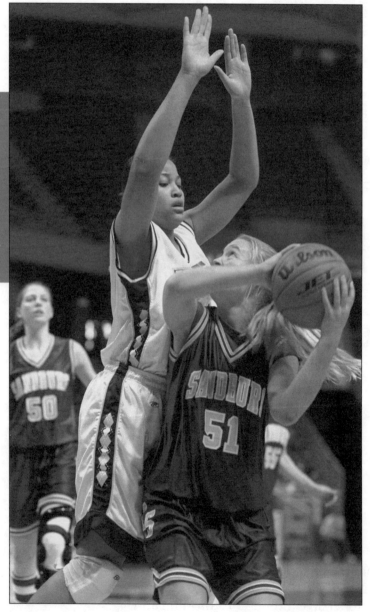

Strength training is the key to better jumping ability.

Basketball, Volleyball, and Netball

Although there are some differences in the jumping actions involved in basketball, volleyball, and netball, athletes use the same major muscle groups in all vertical jumps. Both single-leg and double-leg takeoffs are powered by the calf muscles of the lower leg, the quadriceps and hamstring muscles of the thigh, and the gluteal muscles of the hip. The shoulder muscles (deltoids) also contribute to the jumping action by producing a powerful upward thrust, which is important in two-foot takeoffs.

You can best condition the calf muscles (gastrocnemius and soleus) with standard heel raises, performed with dumbbells, barbells, or machines. Whatever equipment you use, you will achieve better results with full-range ankle movements, facilitated by standing on a step or stable wooden block that permits the heels to drop lower than the toes. Also, you attain more involvement of the large gastrocnemius muscle when you perform heel raises from a straight-leg rather than a bent-knee position.

Although the machine leg extension, leg curl, and leg press should provide plenty of conditioning for the quadriceps and hamstring muscles, the dumbbell lunge offers a more ballistic alternative that will positively impact jumping actions.

Because the hip extensors play a major role in jumping, we recommend that you address these muscles in the training program. The leg press and squat provide progressive resistance exercise for the hamstrings and gluteal muscles that produce hip extension.

Strong shoulder muscles generate powerful upward arm swings that assist in jumping movements. To enhance deltoid development, we suggest a set of machine lateral raises followed almost immediately by a set of machine overhead presses. This double hit on the deltoids is called pre-exhaustion training (two successive exercises for the same muscle group) and is useful for improving muscle strength and endurance. A similar free-weight combination is the dumbbell lateral raise followed by the dumbbell overhead press. We also recommend squat tosses, underhand throws, and lunge passes with medicine balls for increasing power production in the upper body.

Because these sports require significant wrist and forearm strength for proper ball-handling technique, use the super-forearm machine or perform wrist rollers on a homemade pipe, rope, and weight-plate apparatus to strengthen these muscles (see chapter 5 for description and illustration of the wrist roller exercise).

Dance and Figure Skating

Although there are obvious differences between jumping in a dance studio or in an ice rink, the movement patterns and muscle actions are similar. We therefore group these two highly artistic physical activities together for specialized strength training. Although it is not possible to safely or successfully duplicate these dynamic and complex jumping events in the weight room, it may be helpful to add some targeted exercises that directly address the contributing muscle groups.

For the calf muscles of the lower leg, full-range heel raises with machines, barbells, or dumbbells should be most effective. To maximize strength in both the gastrocnemius and soleus muscles of the calf, perform heel raises in a straight-leg rather than a bent-knee position.

Unlike jumping sports in which athletes use carefully designed and highly supportive footwear, dancers and skaters land on hard surfaces with little shoe or skate cushioning to absorb the landing forces. Fortunately, there is a simple but effective exercise for strengthening the front (anterior tibial) muscles of the lower leg to reduce the risk of shin splints, stress fractures, and ankle injuries. The toe raise exercise described in chapter 5 requires only a shoestring and small weight plate to round out lower-leg conditioning.

In addition to leg extensions, leg curls, and leg presses, dancers and skaters who have access to machines should include the hip adduction and hip abduction exercises. These muscles (inner and outer thigh) participate in the numerous lateral movements that characterize most dance and figure-skating performances. It is more difficult to condition these muscles with free weights, but you can use side lunges for this purpose. You should also perform standard lunges to strengthen the quadriceps, hamstrings, and gluteal muscles largely responsible for all jumping actions. Lunges are safer when you perform them holding dumbbells in each hand than with a barbell across the shoulders. Because hip extension is important in dance and skating jumps, be sure to include squats or leg presses for the hamstrings and gluteal muscles.

Most figure-skating jumps and many dance moves require midair turns that athletes accomplish using the midsection, torso, and shoulder muscles. You can enhance the turning actions by using the rotary torso machine to strengthen the external and internal oblique muscles on the sides of the midsection. Diagonal trunk curls serve the same purpose, although without the benefit of progressive resistance.

Overhead presses and pullovers should help jump turns as well as postural stability and upper-body presentation. Overhead presses work the shoulder and triceps muscles, whereas pullovers address the latissimus dorsi muscles of the upper back. You can perform both exercises with machines or dumbbells. If you need more emphasis on the shoulder muscles, do a set of lateral raises (machine or dumbbells) following the pullovers. Dancers and figure skaters should also perform medicine ball exercises such as lunge passes to develop power in the upper and lower extremities.

Applying Jumping Sports Exercise Programs

The sport-specific exercise programs that we have designed for basketball, volleyball, netball, dance, and figure skating emphasize the muscles responsible for the jumping actions inherent in these activities (see appendixes A and B). Of course, there are differences between one-foot jumps in basketball and two-foot jumps in volleyball, as well as between dance jumps on wooden floors and skating jumps on ice. Nonetheless, the jumping similarities far outweigh the differences, and the suggested training exercises should be helpful for enhancing jumping performance in these sports. Remember that we are not trying to imitate actual jumping movements with heavy weights. This would be both difficult and dangerous. Instead, our intent is to condition all the major muscle groups for the purpose of muscle balance and to provide additional training for the muscles that contribute most to jumping power.

Generally, the medicine ball, machine, and free-weight training protocols produce excellent results with one to three sets of each exercise. On the strength exercises, always begin with high repetitions (10 to 15 per set) and progress gradually to medium repetitions (8 to 12 per set). Young athletes who are well conditioned may then work with fewer repetitions (6 to 10 per set), but it is not advisable to use heavy weight loads (5 or fewer repetitions) for sport conditioning. Perform 6 to 10 repetitions per set on the power exercises, and increase the speed of the exercise movements before you increase the weight of the medicine ball. Because the movement speed is fundamental to developing power, don't use a heavy medicine ball for the power exercises.

Because jumping sports place a great deal of stress on both the power-producing muscles and the impact-absorbing muscles, young athletes do not want to overtrain in the weight room. Try to complete three weekly workouts during preseason preparation, but two training sessions per week should be enough when competition begins. Remember that strength building requires ample recovery time for the muscles to respond positively and productively to the training exercises. Fortunately, our research indicates that young people make excellent strength gains on a twice-a-week workout schedule.

Regardless of the strength-training system you select for young athletes, be sure to provide plenty of instruction, supervision, and reinforcement to ensure safe exercise experiences, successful training outcomes, and positive attitudes in all participants. Remember that youth strength training is a team activity.

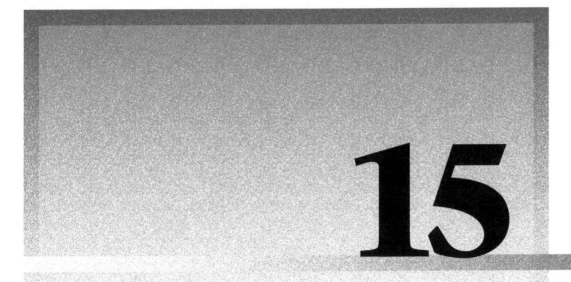

15

Striking Sports: Baseball, Softball, Tennis, Hockey, Golf

The sports of baseball, softball, tennis, hockey, and golf have many differences, mostly related to inherent movement patterns. For example, baseball and softball require sprinting ability to successfully run the bases, tennis is characterized by lateral movements, hockey may be played on turf or on ice, and golf is strictly a stand-in-place sport. Nonetheless, all these sports share the component of striking a ball or puck. Even though the horizontal swinging action of a baseball or softball bat and tennis racket differs from the vertical swinging action of a hockey stick and golf club, the mechanics for developing striking force are the same.

Power production for all striking actions is generated by the large muscles of the legs and hips, transferred through the rotational muscles of the midsection, accelerated by the shoulder joint muscles of the upper body, and applied to the striking implement through the arms. Perfectly synchronized and properly executed striking actions are the result of a highly coordinated and complex series of movements that build on each other to maximize force output and swinging speed. You can use power exercises with medicine balls within a range of motion that mimics your swing. Throwing exercises and movements that require rotation are appropriate for young athletes who play striking sports. Medicine ball lunge passes, side passes, and single-arm throws improve power production in the striking muscles.

You can best develop the precise movement sequencing and summation of forces that produce home run baseball swings and hole-in-one golf drives through repeated practice of these skills. However, the best way to develop the muscle strength that provides the power for these swinging actions is through sensible application of resistance exercise. Beginning with a sound strength- and power-training program that addresses all major muscle groups in a balanced manner, the next step involves specific exercises to better condition the striking muscles. These include the quadriceps, hamstring, hip adductor, hip abductor, and gluteal muscles of the lower body; the abdominal, low-back, and oblique muscles of the midsection; the pectoralis major, latissimus dorsi, and deltoid muscles of the upper body; and the triceps and forearm muscles of the arms. In addition, strong neck muscles are essential for head stability during swinging movements, and well-conditioned forearm muscles are important for control of the striking implement.

Because striking actions involve so many muscles, we suggest adding exercises that use two or more of the target muscle groups. For example, leg presses and squats work the quadriceps, hamstring, and gluteal muscles together. Likewise, medicine ball training works the upper extremities, lower extremities, and trunk muscles simultaneously.

Baseball, Softball, and Tennis

The horizontal striking actions in the baseball swings, softball swings, and tennis drives (forehand and backhand) are similar and derive power from essentially the same muscle groups. Therefore, we present the recommended strength-training exercises for these three sports together.

All horizontal striking movements are initiated by the large muscles of the legs and hips, and are characterized by a powerful hip thrust that transfers weight from the rear leg to the front leg. Although most leg muscles contribute to this explosive action, the hip adductor muscles of the inner thigh and the hip abductor muscles of the outer thigh are key players. Consequently, consider conditioning these muscles on the hip adduction and hip abduction machines if available or performing side lunges with dumbbells.

The torquing action of the midsection muscles transfer the forces produced by the lower body to the upper body. Although the low back and abdominals participate in this power pass, the oblique muscles are largely responsible for the transfer of forces. The best exercise for strengthening the

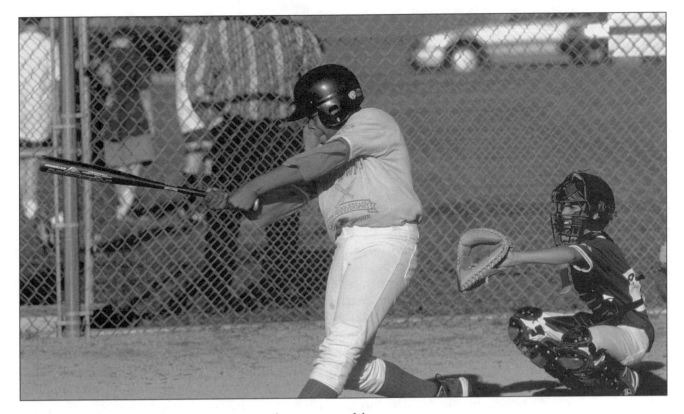

Conditioned striking muscles are stronger and more powerful.

internal and external obliques on both sides of the midsection is the rotary torso machine. If this exercise is not accessible, the diagonal trunk curl is an effective alternative for conditioning the abdominal and oblique muscles together.

The sequential movements of hip thrust and midsection rotation lead to the final phases of the striking action, shoulder rotation, and arm swing. The major upper-body muscles, namely the pectoralis major (chest), latissimus dorsi (upper back), and deltoids (shoulders), accomplish shoulder rotation and arm swing. Powerful contraction of the triceps muscles produce the arm extension movement that culminates the forces in batting and backhand drives. Incline presses (machine or free weights) are ideal for working the pectoralis major, deltoids, and triceps together. Bar dips also involve the pectoralis major, triceps, and deltoid muscles simultaneously.

The shoulder extension action of the tennis serve uses the latissimus dorsi muscles, which are targeted in pullovers (machine or dumbbell) and chin-ups. You can develop grip strength on the super-forearm machine or by performing wrist rollers with a simple pipe, rope, and weight-plate apparatus. This exercise is described and illustrated in chapter 5.

Head stability is essential for maintaining eye focus on a speeding ball, which is why we advise athletes in eye-hand coordination activities (baseball, softball, tennis, hockey, and golf) to perform neck conditioning exercises. For overall neck strengthening it is hard to beat the four-way neck machine. This resistance device addresses the extensor (rear), flexor (front), and lateral flexor (side) muscles of the neck safely and effectively. Although not as comprehensive, the dumbbell

STRIKING SPORTS

shrug is an excellent exercise for the upper trapezius muscle in the rear neck and upper-back area.

Hockey and Golf

The vertical striking actions in hockey and golf swings have several similarities and involve the same muscle groups for power production. For these reasons, the sample strength-training program should enhance striking performance in both sports.

Vertical striking movements derive most of their force from the large muscles of the legs and hips. Like horizontal swings, the powerful hip thrust that shifts weight from the rear leg to the front leg initiates the striking action. Although there is plenty of quadriceps, hamstring, and gluteal involvement, the hip adductor and hip abductor muscles of the inner and outer thigh are largely responsible for the rapid weight transfer and force development. The strength-training program should therefore include machine hip adduction and hip abduction if possible. In the absence of these machines, you can perform side lunges with dumbbells to address these important muscle groups.

Power generated in the lower body must pass to the upper body as efficiently as possible. The torquing action of the midsection muscles accomplishes and accelerates this. The low back and abdominals contribute to the force transfer, but the oblique muscles on the sides of the midsection are key players in this phase of the swing. You can use the rotary torso machine or diagonal trunk curl to strengthen both the internal and external obliques, along with the abdominal muscles.

The next phase of the hockey and golf swing is a diagonal action of the upper body and arms as they drive the stick or club downward and forward as forcefully as possible. This is a complex movement pattern, especially for the large arc golf swing. The essential power-producing muscles include the pectoralis major (chest), latissimus dorsi (upper back), deltoids (shoulders), and triceps (rear arm). Use strength exercises that address several of these muscles simultaneously, such as chest presses (pectoralis major, deltoids, triceps), overhead presses (deltoids, triceps), and bar dips (pectoralis major, triceps, deltoids). Also perform side passes with medicine balls, as they permit acceleration throughout the range of movement. You can use your imagination to modify medicine ball exercises to meet your sport-specific needs.

Strong forearm muscles can ensure a secure, yet relaxed grip on the stick or club, and therefore enhance control of the striking implement. The super-forearm machine provides comprehensive conditioning of the forearm muscles. If this device is unavailable, you can perform wrist rollers by winding and unwinding a weighted rope around a pipe as described in chapter 5.

To strike a ball or moving puck with precision and accuracy, you must firmly fix eye focus throughout the swinging movement. You can facilitate this by a stable head position made possible through strong neck muscles. The four-way neck machine is ideal for overall neck conditioning, as it can strengthen the extensor (rear), flexor (front), and lateral flexor (side) muscles of the neck progressively. The safest free-weight alternative is the dumbbell shrug, which targets the upper trapezius muscle in the rear neck and upper-back area.

Applying Striking Sports Exercise Programs

To be sure, success in the sports of baseball, softball, tennis, hockey, and golf is closely related to the athlete's ability to strike the ball. Although you can improve the striking action through supervised skill practice, performance power largely depends on muscle conditioning. The sample strength- and power-training programs presented in this chapter address all major muscle groups to ensure balanced muscle development. In addition, they include several exercises that target the muscles most prominent in the striking movements (see appendixes A and B). However, you can adjust these training protocols for each athlete, meaning that you can add, eliminate, or substitute exercises based on individual needs, equipment accessibility, time restraints, and conditioning objectives.

In general, begin with the medicine ball power exercises; then perform the strength-building exercises, progressing from large to small muscle groups. Start with the lower body, then upper body, arms, midsection, neck, and forearms. One to three sets of each exercise should be sufficient on the medicine ball, free-weight, and machine exercises. On free weights and machines, always begin with low weight loads and high repetitions; then gradually progress to higher weight loads and lower repetitions. For example, use an initial training protocol of 10 to 15 repetitions per set, then increase the resistance to permit 8 to 12 repetitions, and finally work with higher weight loads for 6 to 10 repetitions per set. It is neither necessary nor desirable for young athletes to train with five or fewer repetitions per set, as heavy weight loads increase the risk of injury. Perform 6 to 10 repetitions per set on the medicine ball exercises, and increase the speed of the exercise movements before you increase the weight of the ball.

Striking is a high-velocity movement that results from powerful muscle contractions. However, striking actions with a bat, racket, stick, or club are much different from similar actions performed with heavy resistance. Due to increased injury potential and skill interference, do not perform any striking action with weights or resistance devices other than medicine balls that you can release at the end of the movement. Perform all strength-building exercises with controlled movement speed through a full range of joint motion. This maximizes muscle involvement and minimizes the role of momentum. Limit fast movement speeds to medicine ball throws.

The athlete's training frequency may vary depending on the conditioning phase. For example, three training sessions per week may be effective during preseason preparation, but two workouts per week may be better tolerated during the competitive period. Remember that muscles require adequate recovery time to build strength levels, and in-season activities may interfere with muscle-building processes. Fortunately, our studies show two strength-training sessions per week are almost as productive as three strength workouts per week.

Most young athletes look forward to power and strength training when you conduct it sensibly in a supervised setting. Keep in mind that good coaching is as important in the weight room as on the athletic field. Competent instruction, sincere encouragement, and positive reinforcement are key factors in successful strength-training experiences.

STRIKING SPORTS

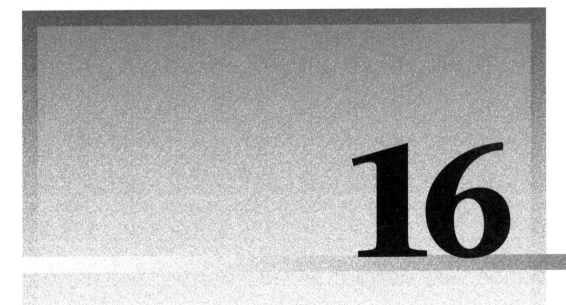

Endurance Sports: Soccer, Field Hockey, Lacrosse, Cross Country, Swimming

The sports of soccer, field hockey, lacrosse, cross country, and swimming are endurance activities. With the exceptions of goaltenders and sprint swimmers, athletes in these sports are usually in motion. The continual action requires high levels of cardiovascular and muscular endurance for successful and sustained performance.

Although these aerobic activities are less dependent on muscle strength than power sports, strength training should be a major component in the conditioning programs. First, because every physical action (sprinting, running, swimming, etc.) uses a certain percentage of maximum muscle strength, a stronger athlete has an advantage over a weaker athlete. This is especially true in sports such as soccer, field hockey, and lacrosse, which are characterized by stop-and-go activity and require intermittent acceleration and deceleration.

Second, due to the repetitive nature of endurance sports, these athletes have a high incidence of overuse injuries. Strength training improves muscle balance and increases musculoskeletal resistance to repetitive stress. This is important for cross country runners and swimmers who perform the same movement patterns thousands of times every practice session. Remember our strength-trained cross country team that won four consecutive New England championships and experienced only one injury during those years (see chapter 12).

The sports of soccer, field hockey, and lacrosse have similar conditioning requirements, and we group them together for strength training. Cross country running is a lower-body activity, whereas swimming emphasizes the upper-body muscles. Therefore, we present different strength-training programs to specifically address the conditioning needs of runners and swimmers. Similarly, we suggest different power-training medicine ball exercises for these athletes.

Soccer, Field Hockey, and Lacrosse

In these field sports, athletes sprint, change direction, and sprint again. The muscles largely responsible for these rapid accelerations and decelerations are the quadriceps, hamstrings, gluteals, and calves. Basic exercises for strengthening these muscles are the barbell squat, machine leg press, and heel raise. Both the barbell squat and machine leg press work the quadriceps, hamstrings, and gluteal muscles simultaneously. Key power exercises for improving speed and quickness in the lower extremities are the medicine ball squat toss and lunge pass.

Heel raises produce the same effect on the calf muscles (gastrocnemius and soleus) whether performed with dumbbells, barbells, or machines. For best overall calf conditioning, do heel raises from a straight-leg rather than a bent-knee position.

Because soccer, field hockey, and lacrosse involve many lateral movements, the recommended training program addresses the inner- and outer-thigh muscles. The hip adduction and hip abduction machines directly target these muscles, and the dumbbell side lunge is an effective free-weight alternative.

The striking actions in field hockey and the throwing movements in lacrosse require efficient force transfer from the legs to the upper body. The midsection muscles accomplish this, especially the internal and external obliques that surround the sides. The rotary torso machine provides an excellent means for strengthening the oblique muscles, but diagonal trunk curls are also productive for this purpose.

The kicking action in soccer involves the hip flexor muscles. A simple and effective means for strengthening these muscles is the hanging-knee raise performed from dip bars.

ENDURANCE SPORTS

Although upper-body strength may not be of paramount importance, all three sports can benefit from well-conditioned triceps muscles. Soccer throw-ins, field hockey swings, and lacrosse stick throws are triceps actions that you can strengthen by bar dips (machine or body weight) and overhead throws with medicine balls. To perform the overhead throw exercise, hold the medicine ball behind your head with your elbows bent, then throw the ball as far as possible.

Grip strength is advantageous for stick control in field hockey and lacrosse. The super-forearm machine works all muscles involved in gripping and wrist actions. If this equipment is unavailable, wrist rollers offer a good alternative, using a pipe, rope, and weight-plate apparatus. This exercise is described and illustrated in chapter 5.

Strong neck muscles are essential for heading a soccer ball safely and successfully. We recommend the four-way neck machine that works the extensor (rear), flexor (front), and lateral flexor (side) muscles of the neck. An effective free-weight exercise for the neck extensor muscles is the dumbbell shrug.

Cross Country

Although cross country and track distance runners are not power athletes, they can benefit from an appropriate strength- and power-training program. Perhaps the major advantages for strength-trained runners is the reduced risk of overuse injuries so prevalent in this sport. Training all major muscle groups to a high level of strength fitness ensures balanced muscle development and greater shock absorption ability. Although you can meet this conditioning objective by the general strength-training programs presented in chapter 12, there are some specific exercises to enhance running ability. This section presents these exercises and places them in sample machine and free-weight training protocols for distance runners.

Without question, cross country running is a cardiovascular activity mostly involving the heart, lungs, and legs. At least that is how many people perceive this sport. In reality, the midsection and upper-body muscles contribute much to successful distance running. The continuous and high-volume breathing required during hard runs and races places considerable stress on the midsection muscles. It is therefore advisable for runners to do strengthening exercises for the abdominal and oblique muscles.

Every running stride is counterbalanced by a matching arm action, so the left leg and right arm always move in a synchronized pattern, as do the right leg and left arm. A strong upper body is therefore a great advantage when the legs start to tire, as an unrelenting arm drive will keep the legs moving in matching rhythm.

Another important conditioning concern for runners is the upper-back, shoulder, and neck area. When this part of the body begins to fatigue and tighten up, the race is over.

With these points in mind, runners should add the following exercises to their general strength-training program. For midsection conditioning, make sure every workout includes the rotary torso machine or diagonal trunk curls for the oblique muscles that surround the sides. Hanging-knee raises from dip bars address the abdominal and hip flexor muscles involved in every running stride.

The shoulder and neck muscles are the most active upper-body groups during distance runs. Use lateral raises (machine or dumbbells) followed by overhead presses (machine or dumbbells) for emphasis on the deltoid muscles. You can comprehensively strengthen the neck area on the four-way neck machine. If this apparatus is unavailable, condition the neck extensor muscles by performing the dumbbell shrug exercise.

Because many runners experience lower-leg injuries such as shin splints and stress fractures, be sure to include a strengthening exercise for the shin muscles to maintain muscle balance in the lower leg. A simple but successful means for training the anterior tibial (shin) muscles is toe raises using a shoestring and weight plate (see chapter 5).

Swimming

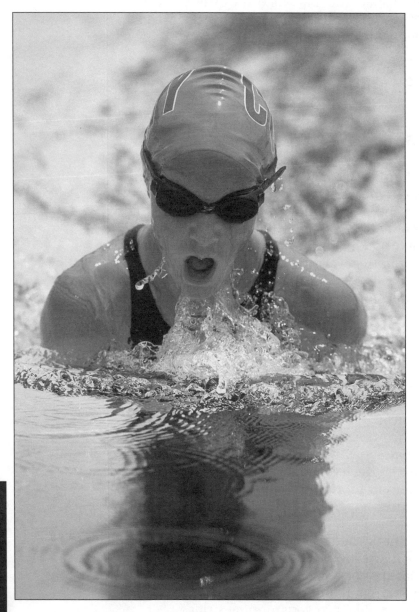

Swimmers can benefit from strength training through increased endurance and stronger bodies.

Like track, swimming includes a variety of events from short to long duration. All swimmers can benefit from strength and power training, and those who do distance events are no exception. Distance swimmers are similar to cross country runners in terms of aerobic energy requirements, and both activities require a well-conditioned cardiovascular system for successful participation. However, you can enhance both running and swimming performance through a sensible program of strength training that increases muscle strength and endurance. Swimmers may also reduce their risk of overuse injuries by developing balanced strength, especially around the shoulder joint.

Unlike most other sports, swimming takes place in the isokinetic environment of water. In isokinetic exercise, the movement force you give determines the resistance force you receive. For example, if you give a light push with your hand against the water you will encounter a low resistance from the water. If you give a hard push against the water you will encounter a high resistance from the water. Although you must work harder to swim faster, the increase in speed is not proportional to the increase in effort. Because every swimming stroke requires a certain percentage of maximum strength, a stronger swimmer is definitely a better swimmer. Basically, muscle strength is almost as important as body build and stroke mechanics for competitive swimming success.

An analysis of the muscles most relevant to swimming performance shows that the primary force producers for the arm-pulling action are the upper-back (latissimus dorsi) muscles. You can target these muscles by machine pullovers or dumbbell pullovers, as well as by chin-ups. The chest (pectoralis major) muscles also contribute to pulling power, and you can appropriately strengthen them with bar dips.

The shoulder (deltoid) muscles are most active during the recovery phase of the arm stroke, when the hand is out of the water. Lateral raises, performed on a machine or with dumbbells, are highly effective for deltoid conditioning. For greater shoulder emphasis, you can follow lateral raises by overhead presses (machine or dumbbells), which work the deltoids and triceps simultaneously.

The leg action for flutter kicking is largely produced by the quadriceps, hamstrings, and gluteal muscles. Machine leg presses and barbell squats address all these muscles together and should be staple exercises in swimmers' training programs. We also recommend hanging-knee raises performed on dip bars for powerful kicking movements. Of course, breaststrokers should also perform hip adduction and hip abduction exercises for the inner- and outer-thigh muscles that are prominent in this swimming event.

The crawl stroke requires rhythmic turning of the torso and head, which depends on strong midsection and neck muscles. If available, use the rotary torso machine to strengthen the oblique muscles that surround the midsection and the four-way neck machine to condition all areas of the neck (extensors, flexors, and lateral flexors). If these machines are not accessible, substitute diagonal trunk curls for the rectus abdominis and oblique muscles, and dumbbell shrugs for the neck extensor muscles.

Due to the high incidence of shoulder rotator cuff injuries among swimmers, their strength-training program should include external and internal rotation exercises on the rotary shoulder machine, with a dumbbell or on a pulley apparatus as shown in the photos. By strengthening this vulnerable aspect of shoulder joint movement, you should greatly reduce the risk of rotator cuff problems.

Applying Endurance Sports Exercise Programs

The sample sport-specific strength-training programs are merely suggestions, and coaches may make appropriate changes consistent with their conditioning objectives, time limitations, equipment resources, and facility factors. There is no program that is perfect for all athletes, and you must adapt the strength-training protocols to individual needs and abilities.

Nonetheless, endurance sports have similar requirements for improving muscle endurance and thereby enhancing athletic performance. Generally, participants in endurance activities respond better to high repetitions with low weight loads than to low repetitions with high weight loads. Therefore, begin with 15 to 20 repetitions per set, and progress to 10 to 15 repetitions per set. As a rule, endurance athletes should train with resistances that they can lift at least 10 times in good form.

ENDURANCE SPORTS

Due to their emphasis on sustained muscle activity, these athletes may want to perform two or three sets of each exercise in close succession. Although multiple sets are not necessary for strength development, they may be helpful for increasing muscle endurance (see appendixes A and B for appropriate exercises for endurance sports).

Endurance athletes may also want to strength train more frequently than power athletes. However, they should not do more than every-other-day strength workouts during the off-season. Because many endurance athletes overtrain, they should cut back to two strength sessions per week during the competitive period. This training frequency is more than sufficient to build and maintain strength for enhanced performance and reduced injury risk.

Training with high repetitions is sometimes associated with fast and short exercise movements to complete the set quickly. However, endurance athletes should use controlled movement speed and full movement range on every repetition. This produces effective muscle tension and develops muscle endurance, which are primary objectives of the training program. Performing fast and short repetitions emphasizes momentum more than muscle and may increase the risk of injury. The only exercises that you should do quickly are the medicine ball throws in which you can accelerate and release the resistance. Endurance athletes should perform one to two sets of 6 to 10 repetitions on all power exercises.

Endurance athletes are typically dedicated and hard-working individuals who may overtrain if not supervised carefully. Therefore, the coach should be present during every strength-training session to ensure proper exercise form and appropriate exercise effort. Also, it is hard to overemphasize encouragement and positive reinforcement to young athletes during strength-training workouts.

Appendix A

Free Weights

Free Weight Exercises

	BB squat	DB step-up	DB lunge	DB side lunge	BB heel raise	DB heel raise	Toe raise	BB bench press	DB incline press	DB pullover	DB one-arm row	DB lateral raise	DB overhead press	DB biceps curl	DB incline biceps curl
Baseball	✓	✓		✓				✓	✓	✓	✓			✓	
Basketball	✓	✓	✓		✓			✓			✓	✓	✓	✓	
Cross country	✓	✓					✓	✓			✓	✓	✓		
Dance	✓	✓		✓		✓	✓	✓		✓	✓	✓	✓		✓
Distance running	✓	✓					✓	✓			✓	✓	✓	✓	
Field hockey	✓	✓		✓	✓			✓	✓		✓		✓	✓	
Figure skating	✓	✓		✓		✓	✓	✓		✓	✓	✓	✓		✓
Football	✓		✓		✓			✓	✓		✓				✓
Golf	✓	✓		✓				✓	✓	✓	✓		✓		✓
Gymnastics	✓		✓		✓			✓			✓		✓	✓	
Hockey	✓	✓		✓				✓	✓	✓	✓		✓		✓
Lacrosse	✓	✓		✓	✓			✓			✓		✓	✓	
Netball	✓	✓	✓		✓			✓			✓	✓	✓	✓	
Rugby	✓	✓	✓		✓			✓	✓		✓				✓
Soccer	✓	✓		✓	✓			✓			✓		✓	✓	
Softball	✓	✓		✓				✓	✓	✓	✓			✓	
Swimming	✓	✓					✓	✓		✓	✓	✓	✓	✓	
Tennis	✓	✓		✓				✓	✓	✓	✓			✓	
Track and field	✓		✓		✓			✓	✓		✓				✓
Volleyball	✓	✓	✓		✓			✓			✓	✓	✓	✓	
Wrestling	✓		✓					✓			✓		✓	✓	

Note. MB = medicine ball; BB = barbell; DB = dumbbell.

DB triceps kickback	DB triceps overhead extension	Chin-up	Bar dip	Prone back raise	Trunk curl	Diagonal trunk curl	Hanging-knee raise	DB shrug	DB shoulder external rotation	DB shoulder internal rotation	DB wrist curl	DB wrist extension	Wrist roller	MB squat toss	MB lunge pass	MB chest pass	MB sidei pass	MB underhand throw	MB single arm throw
✓		✓	✓	✓		✓		✓					✓		✓		✓		✓
✓				✓	✓								✓	✓	✓			✓	
✓		✓	✓	✓		✓	✓	✓						✓	✓	✓			
	✓			✓		✓								✓	✓			✓	
✓		✓	✓	✓		✓	✓	✓						✓	✓	✓			
	✓	✓	✓	✓		✓							✓	✓	✓	✓			
	✓			✓		✓							✓	✓				✓	
✓		✓	✓	✓	✓			✓					✓	✓		✓		✓	
✓		✓	✓	✓		✓		✓					✓		✓		✓	✓	
	✓	✓	✓	✓		✓	✓				✓	✓	✓		✓			✓	
✓	✓	✓	✓	✓		✓		✓					✓		✓		✓	✓	
	✓	✓	✓	✓		✓							✓	✓	✓	✓			
✓				✓	✓								✓	✓	✓			✓	
✓		✓	✓	✓	✓			✓					✓	✓		✓		✓	
	✓	✓	✓	✓		✓	✓	✓						✓	✓	✓			
✓		✓	✓	✓		✓		✓					✓		✓		✓		✓
✓		✓	✓	✓		✓		✓	✓	✓			✓	✓		✓			
✓		✓	✓	✓		✓		✓					✓		✓		✓		✓
✓		✓	✓	✓		✓	✓				✓	✓	✓		✓			✓	
✓				✓	✓								✓	✓	✓			✓	
	✓	✓	✓	✓		✓		✓					✓	✓		✓		✓	

Appendix B

Weight Machines

Weight Machine Exercises

Sport	Leg press	Leg extension	Leg curl	Hip abduction	Hip adduction	Heel raise	Toe raise	Chest press	Pullover	Seated row	Lateral raise	Overhead press	Biceps curl
Baseball	✓	✓	✓	✓	✓			✓	✓	✓		✓	✓
Basketball	✓	✓	✓			✓		✓		✓	✓	✓	✓
Cross country	✓	✓	✓				✓	✓		✓	✓	✓	✓
Dance	✓	✓	✓	✓	✓	✓		✓	✓	✓	✓	✓	✓
Distance running	✓	✓	✓				✓	✓		✓	✓	✓	✓
Field hockey	✓	✓	✓	✓	✓	✓		✓		✓		✓	✓
Figure skating	✓	✓	✓	✓	✓	✓		✓	✓	✓	✓	✓	✓
Football	✓			✓	✓	✓		✓		✓		✓	✓
Golf	✓	✓	✓	✓	✓			✓	✓	✓		✓	✓
Gymnastics	✓	✓	✓			✓		✓		✓		✓	✓
Hockey	✓	✓	✓	✓	✓			✓	✓	✓		✓	✓
Lacrosse	✓	✓	✓	✓	✓	✓		✓		✓		✓	✓
Netball	✓	✓	✓			✓		✓		✓	✓	✓	✓
Rugby	✓			✓	✓	✓		✓		✓		✓	✓
Soccer	✓	✓	✓	✓	✓	✓		✓		✓		✓	✓
Softball	✓	✓	✓	✓	✓			✓	✓	✓		✓	✓
Swimming	✓	✓	✓	✓	✓			✓	✓	✓	✓	✓	✓
Tennis	✓	✓	✓	✓	✓			✓	✓	✓		✓	✓
Track and field	✓	✓	✓			✓		✓		✓		✓	✓
Volleyball	✓	✓	✓			✓		✓		✓	✓	✓	✓
Wrestling	✓	✓	✓	✓	✓			✓		✓		✓	✓

Note: MB = medicine ball.

Triceps extension	Weight-assisted chin-up	Weight-assisted bar dip	Low-back extension	Abdominal curl	Rotary torso	Hanging-knee raise	Neck extension	Neck flexion	Rotary shoulder	Super forearm	MB squat toss	MB lunge pass	MB chest pass	MB underhand throw	MB side pass	MB single arm throw
✓	✓	✓	✓	✓	✓		✓	✓		✓		✓			✓	✓
✓			✓	✓						✓	✓	✓		✓		
✓	✓	✓	✓	✓	✓	✓	✓	✓			✓	✓	✓			
✓			✓	✓	✓						✓	✓		✓		
✓	✓	✓	✓	✓	✓	✓	✓	✓			✓	✓	✓			
✓	✓	✓	✓	✓	✓	✓	✓	✓		✓	✓	✓	✓			
✓			✓	✓	✓						✓	✓		✓		
✓	✓	✓	✓	✓			✓	✓		✓	✓		✓	✓		
✓	✓	✓	✓	✓	✓		✓	✓		✓		✓		✓	✓	
✓	✓	✓	✓	✓	✓	✓				✓	✓		✓	✓		
✓	✓		✓	✓	✓		✓	✓		✓		✓			✓	
✓	✓	✓	✓	✓	✓	✓	✓	✓		✓	✓	✓	✓			
✓			✓	✓						✓	✓	✓		✓		
✓	✓	✓	✓	✓			✓	✓		✓	✓		✓	✓		
✓	✓	✓	✓	✓	✓	✓	✓	✓		✓	✓	✓	✓			
✓	✓	✓	✓	✓			✓	✓		✓		✓			✓	✓
✓	✓	✓	✓	✓	✓		✓	✓	✓		✓	✓	✓			
✓	✓	✓	✓	✓	✓		✓	✓		✓		✓			✓	✓
✓	✓	✓	✓	✓	✓	✓				✓	✓		✓	✓		
✓			✓	✓						✓	✓	✓	✓		✓	
✓	✓	✓	✓	✓	✓	✓		✓	✓		✓	✓	✓		✓	✓

Index

A

age-group strength programs 137-151

B

baseball, softball, and tennis
    exercises 182-184
    target muscles 182-184
basketball, volleyball, and netball
    exercises 178-179
    target muscles 178-179
body-weight exercises
    about 122
    advantages and disadvantages 121
    lower body, upper body, and midsection 122-134
    summary 135
body-weight exercises, lower-body
    heel raise 125
    squat 123
    walking lunge 124
body-weight exercises, midsection
    back extension 134
    hanging-knee raise 130
    kneeling-trunk extension 132
    pelvic tilt 131
    prone back raise 133
    trunk curl and diagonal trunk curl 129
body-weight exercises, upper-body
    bar dip 128
    chin-up 127
    push-up 126

C

carbohydrates
    about 30
    glycemic index, high and low 30
children, understanding
    adequate recovery 23
    knowledgeable adults as strength-training instructors 23

strength training as year-round conditioning program 23
cords and balls
    about 93-94
    medicine ball exercises 105-119
    rubber cord exercises 95-104
    summary 119
    training with 94
cross country
    exercises 189-190
    target muscles 189-190

D

dance and figure skating
    exercises 179-180
    target muscles 179-180
dumbbell exercises (10- to 12-year-olds) 148*t*

E

eating for strength
    basics for healthy eating 31
    carbohydrates 30
    children's nutritional needs 28-29
    fats 34, 35
    fruit 32, 33
    grains 31-32
    meats 33, 34
    milk products 33
    power eating 27-28
    proper nutrition, about 27
    protein requirements 29
    snack foods 30-31
    summary 35
    vegetables 32
    vitamins and minerals 30
    weak nutrition, defined 27
endurance sports
    about 187
    applying endurance sports exercise programs 191-192
    cross country 189-190

soccer, field hockey, and lacrosse 188-189
strength training in conditioning programs 188
swimming 190-191
endurance sports exercise programs, applying
    repetitions and sets, range of 191-192
    supervision, instruction, and encouragement 192
    training frequency 192
equipment, factors to consider when evaluating 11
equipment, using safely
    safe exercise setting 25-26
    safety precautions, following 25
    spotter, teaching proper 26
equipment selection
    beginning exercises 10
    exercise techniques *versus* equipment used 10
exercise programs for general sport conditioning, about 165

F

fats
    fat content of meat 34*t*
    high-fat food consumption 35
    sample exchange units equivalent to one fat serving 35*t*
    saturated and monounsaturated 34
fitness, fundamental
    benefits of 6
    strength-training programs 6
    youths, sport participants, about 5-6
    youths with little physical activity, about 5
football and rugby
    exercises 174-175
    target muscles 174

free-weight exercises
    lower-body exercises 44-51
    safety guidelines 42-43
    sport appropriate 197-199
    upper body exercises 52-69
free-weight exercises-8 stations (13-
    to 15-year-olds) 155t
free-weight exercises-12 stations
    (13- to 15-year-olds) 156t
free weights
    exercises 42-69
    form and technique, teaching 40
    improper exercise technique and
        injury 41
    safe exercise setting 39-40
    spotting techniques,
        demonstrating proper 40-41
    summary 70
    supervision and instruction 41
    teaching exercises, procedures for
        40
    training with 41-42
free weights, training with
    advantages of 42
    barbells and dumbbells, about
        41
    instruction and supervision 42
    weight benches, flat and incline
        41-42
free-weight strength-training
    exercises 148t
fruit
    dried 32
    nutritional value 32
    one serving size 33t
    servings per day 33

G
grains
    about 31
    recommended servings of 32
gymnastics
    exercises 175
    taget muscles 175

H
healthy eating, basics for 31
hockey and golf
    exercises 184
    target muscles 184

J
jog and catch, procedures 106
jumping sports
    about 177-178
    applying jumping sports exercise
        programs 180
    basketball, volleyball, and netball
        178-179
    dance and figure skating 179-
        180
jumping sports exercise programs,
    applying
    instruction, supervision and
        reinforcement 180
    overtraining 180
    repetition range 180

junior builders: 10- to 12-year-olds
    about 145
    free-weight strength-training
        exercises 148
    machine strength-training
        exercises 147t
    strength-training program 146
    training considerations 149-150
    warm-up and cool-down
        components 146

L
lower-body exercises (free weights)
    barbell heel raise 50
    barbell squat 45
    dumbbell heel raise 49
    dumbbell lunge 46
    dumbbell side lunge 47
    dumbbell squat 44
    dumbbell step-up 48
    heel raise 78
    hip abduction 77
    hip adduction 77
    leg curl 76
    leg extension 75
    leg press 74
    toe raise 51
lower-body exercises (weight
    machines)
    heel raise 78
    hip abduction 77
    hip adduction 77
    leg curl 76
    leg extension 75
    leg press 74

M
machine and free-weight strength-
    training exercises (7- to 9-year-
    olds), about 140-141
machine and free-weight strength-
    training exercises (13- to 15-
    year-olds), about 154
machine strength-training exercises
    147t
meats
    fat content of 34t
    nutritional value 33
    one serving size of 34t
    protein per serving 34
medicine ball exercises
    about 105
    power exercises 115-118
    strength exercises 108-114
    warm-up exercises 106-107
    weights and sizes, variety of 105
medicine balls 94
medicine ball warm-up exercises
    around the world 106
    ball march 106
    body stretch 107
    helicopter circles 107
    jog and catch 106
mighty mites: 7-to 9-year-olds
    about 139

machine and free-weight
    strength-training exercises
    140-141
strength-training program 140
training considerations 141-143
warm-up and cool-down
    components 140
milk products
    nutritional value of 33
    servings per day 33
muscles, bones, and connective tissue
    misconceptions 6
    musculoskeletal system, about 6
    strength training benefits for 6

N
nutritional needs, children's
    balance 29
    Food Guide Pyramid, about 28, 28f
    healthy foods, ideas for
        motivating youths to want
        28-29
    role modeling 29
    snacks, low in fat 29

P
power exercises (medicine ball)
    chest pass 117
    lunge pass 116
    side pass 117
    single-arm throw 118
    squat toss 115
    underhand throw 118
power sports
    about 173-174
    applying power sports exercise
        programs 176
    football and rugby 174-175
    gymnastics 175
    medicine ball drills for power
        development 174
    track and field 176
    wrestling 175
power sports exercise programs,
    applying
    muscle recovery 176
    precautions 176
    repetition ranges 176
    sport coaches, importance of
        involvement 176
    training sessions per week 176
power training for general sport
    conditioning
    about 162
    medicine ball, exercises, about
        162, 163
program, prescribed
    Delorme-Watkins training
        protocol 12
    guidelines 11-12
    movement speed, controlled 12
    muscle strength, training
        procedures for increasing 12
    strength workout 13
    training efficiency and exercise
        effectiveness, enhancing 12

program, progressive
  individual abilities, recognizing 26
  program, fresh and challenging 26
program considerations
  adults understanding strength-training principles 11
  children appreciating benefits and risks 11
program design
  interacting with each child 19, 20
  kids workout log 20f
  standard free-weight and machine exercises for major muscle groups 14t
  stretches for young strength trainers 15-18
  stretching and warm-ups 13
  training consistency and rewards 19
  winners and losers atmosphere, avoiding 19
program prescriptions
  about 9
  equipment selection 10
  order and control 10
  personalized programs 9-10
  safe exercise setting 10
  summary 20
  training guidelines 11-20
protein requirements
  servings needed for youths in strength-training programs, examples of 29
  too much, problems with 29

R
readiness
  emotional maturity 7
  overtraining, preventing 7
  program, importance of individualized 7
  workout protocols for children, about 7-8
Rose, George 162
rubber cord exercises
  biceps curl 103
  lateral raise 100
  lat pulldown 101
  leg curl 96
  seated row 102
  seated shoulder press 98
  squat 95
  standing chest press 97
  triceps extension 104
  upright row 99
rubber cords and medicine balls, training with
  adjusting for appropriate amount of stretch 94
  inspecting, what to look for 94
  proper use of 94

S
snack foods
  about 30
  ideas for healthy snacks 31
  sweets, alternatives for 31
soccer, field hockey, and lacrosse
  exercises 188-189
  target muscles 188-189
sport-conditioning programs, general
  about 161-162
  applying strength- and power-training programs 165, 172
  exercise programs for general sport conditioning 165
  Notre Dame High School cross country team strength-training exercises 163t
  overall muscle conditioning, importance of 162
  power training for general sport conditioning 162, 163
  strength training for general sport conditioning 163-165
spotter, requirements of 40-41
strength- and power-training programs, applying
  general conditioning using free weights—advanced 168t
  general conditioning using free weights—beginners 166t
  general conditioning using free weights—intermediate 167t
  general conditioning using resistance machines—advanced 171t
  general conditioning using resistance machines—beginners 169t
  general conditioning using resistance machines—intermediate 170t
  sport conditioning, key to successful 165, 172
strength development 1-36
strength exercises (medicine ball)
  biceps curl 112
  front shoulder raise 109
  front squat 108
  side bend 114
  supine chest press 110
  triceps press 111
  twist and turn 113
strength programs for sports 159-187
strength training for general sport conditioning
  legs 164
  neck 164-165
  trunk 164
  upper arms 164
  upper body 164
strength-training program (7- to 9-year-olds)

effective conditioning 140
youth strength-training guidelines 140
strength-training program (10- to 12-year-olds)
  about 146
  exercises to use 146
strength-training program (13- to 15-year-olds)
  about 152
  equipment, learning and practicing with 152-153
  strength-training protocols with exercise equipment, guidelines for designing 153, 153t, 154
strength training versus weightlifting
  strength training, defined 4-5
  weightlifting, defined 5
stretches for young strength trainers
  calf stretch 18
  certificate of completion 19f
  chest stretch 15
  hamstring stretch 16
  inner-thigh stretch 17
  low-back and hip stretch 17
  quadriceps stretch 18
  triceps and lat stretch 15
  upper-back stretch 16
striking sports
  about 181
  applying striking sports exercise programs 185
  baseball, softball, and tennis 182-184
  hockey and golf 184
  muscle strength, developing 182
  power production 182
striking sports exercise programs, applying
  instruction, supervision, and encouragement 185
  striking action, performing 185
  training protocol, starting 185
swimming
  exercises for strengthening specific muscles 190-191
  isokinetic exercise, about 190-191
  muscles used 190-191

T
teacher, being a
  education as major focus 24
  goal of program, looking beyond 24
  participation, reasons for 24
  role of 23-24
technique and injury prevention, correct
  focus of program 22
  keeping it progressive 26
  safety of program, steps for ensuring 22

summary 26
supervision 21
teaching 23-24
understanding children 23
using equipment safely 25-26
teens of steel: 13- to 15-year-olds
    machine and free-weight strength-training exercises 154
    strength exercise, developmental advantages of 151-152
    strength training and muscle strength, study on 151
    strength-training program 152-153, 154
    training considerations 154, 155, 157
    warm-up and cool-down components 152
track and field
    exercises 176
    target muscles 176
training, readiness for
    about 3
    fundamental fitness 5-6
    getting ready 7-8
    guidelines, about 4
    muscles, bones, and connective tissue 6
    strength training versus weightlifting 4-5
    summary 8
    training guidelines from medical and fitness organizations, about 3-4
training considerations (7-to 9-year-olds)
    appropriate machine and free-weight exercises 141-142
    child-sized weight machines exercises 142t
    dumbbell exercises 143t
    instruction and supervision 142, 143
    proper exercise form 142
training considerations (10- to 12-year-olds)
    body-weight exercises 149
    equipment 149
    supervision, instruction, and encouragement 149-150

training considerations (13- to 15-year-olds)
    advantages 157
    body weight, exercises encouraging teens to handle 154, 155
    elastic bands 155
    free weight exercises—8 stations 155t
    free weight exercises—12 stations 156t
    instruction and supervision 157
    resistance machine exercises—8 stations 157t
    resistance machine exercises—14 stations 158t
training guidelines
    certificate of completion 19f
    equipment 11
    prescribed program 11-13
    program considerations 11, 19, 20
    program design 13-20
    research studies and refinements of 12-13
    standard free-weight and machine exercises for major muscle groups 14t
    stretches for young strength trainers 15-18
training on weight machines
    safe and effective for children, guidelines 72-73
    safety steps before and during exercise sessions 73

U
upper-body exercises (free weights)
    barbell bench press 54
    dumbbell biceps curl 64
    dumbbell chest fly 55
    dumbbell chest press 52
    dumbbell incline biceps curl 64
    dumbbell incline press 53
    dumbbell lateral raise 60
    dumbbell one-arm row 56
    dumbbell overhead press 59
    dumbbell pullover 57
    dumbbell shoulder external rotation 62
    dumbbell shoulder internal rotation 63
    dumbbell shrug 61
    dumbbell triceps kickback 65

dumbbell triceps overhead extension 66
    dumbbell upright row 58
    dumbbell wrist curl 67
    dumbbell wrist extension 68
    wrist roller 69
upper-body exercises (weight machines)
    abdominal curl 87
    biceps curl 86
    chest press 79
    front pulldown 81
    lateral raise 83
    low-back extension 88
    neck extension 90
    neck flexion 90
    overhead press 83
    pullover 82
    rotary shoulder 91
    rotary torso 89
    seated row 80
    super forearm 91
    triceps extension 84
    triceps pressdown 85

V
vegetables
    about 32
    recommended daily servings of 32
vitamins and minerals
    antioxidants 30
    when to take 30

W
weight-machine exercises
    about 73
    lower body 74-78
    sport appropriate 193-195
    upper body 79-91
weight-machine exercises, youth-sized (10- to 12-olds) 147t
weight machines
    advantages of 71
    exercises 73-91
    proper fit, importance of 71-72
    summary 92
    training on 72-73
    youth strength-training equipment, advantages of 72
wrestling
    exercises 175
    target muscles 175

About the Authors

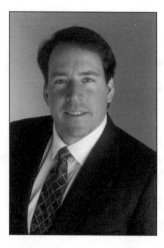

As a leading researcher and practitioner in the area of youth fitness, Avery Faigenbaum, EdD, CSCS, has had years of experience working with children and adolescents in the weight room. He is currently an assistant professor of human performance and fitness at the University of Massachusetts—working as a pediatric exercise scientist as well as fitness practitioner and youth volunteer.

A well-recognized and sought-after speaker, Faigenbaum lectures across the country to sports medicine and fitness organizations. He serves on the editorial boards of the *Strength and Conditioning Journal, Journal of Strength and Conditioning Research,* and *ACSM's Health and Fitness Journal.* Faigenbaum is certified by the NSCA, ACSM, and the United States Weightlifting Association. He was awarded Junior Investigator of the Year by the NCSA in 1999 and was honored with the Hodgkinson Adult Volunteer of the Year by the South Shore YMCA in 1998. He has also been appointed to the Massachusetts Governors Committee on Physical Fitness and Sports and elected to serve as NSCA Massachusetts State Director. Faigenbaum lives in Boston, Massachusetts.

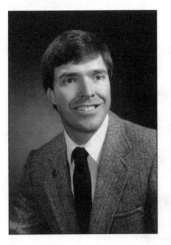

With more than 35 years of experience in strength training as an athlete, coach, teacher, professor, researcher, writer, and speaker, Wayne Westcott, PhD, CSCS, is recognized as a leading authority on fitness. He has served as a strength training consultant for numerous organizations and programs, including Nautilus, the President's Council on Physical Fitness and Sports, the National Sports Performance Association, the International Association of Fitness Professionals (IDEA), the American Council on Exercise, the YMCA of the USA, and the National Youth Sports Safety Foundation. He was awarded the IDEA Lifetime Achievement Award in 1993 and was honored with a Healthy American Fitness Leader Award in 1995.

Westcott is the fitness research director at the South Shore YMCA in Quincy, Massachusetts. He has authored twelve books on strength training, including four with Human Kinetics—*Building Strength and Stamina* (1996), *Strength Training Past 50* (1998), *Strength Training for Seniors* (1999), and *Complete Conditioning for Golf* (1999). He has published more than 400 articles in professional fitness journals and has written a weekly fitness column for one of Boston's largest newspapers since 1986. He has served on the editorial boards of *Prevention, Shape, Men's Health, Fitness, Club Industry, American Fitness Quarterly,* and *Nautilus.* Westcott lives in Abington, Massachusetts, with his wife, Claudia.

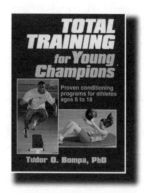
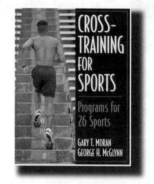
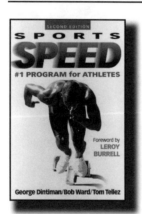